The Type 1/Type 2 Allergy Relief Program

The Type 1/Type 2 Allergy Relief Program

INCLUDING INFORMATION ON:
Testing Procedures
At-Home Self-Treatment
Office, Home, and Vacation Strategies
The Allergy-Obesity Diet
Medical Breakthroughs
Choosing the Right Allergist

Alan S. Levin, M.D., and Merla Zellerbach
Research Assistant—Debra Lynn Dadd

JEREMY P. TARCHER, INC.
Los Angeles
Distributed by Houghton Mifflin Company
Boston

Library of Congress Cataloging in Publication Data

Levin, Alan S.
   The type 1/type 2 allergy relief program.

   Bibliography: p. 215.
   Includes index.
   1. Allergy.   I. Zellerbach, Merla.   II. Dadd, Debra
Lynn.   III. Title.
   RC584.L48 1983   626.97   83-4744
   ISBN 0-87477-328-8 (pbk.)

Copyright © 1983 by Alan S. Levin, M.D., and Merla Zellerbach

Jeremy P. Tarcher, Inc.
9110 Sunset Blvd.
Los Angeles, CA 90069

Design by Tanya Maiboroda

MANUFACTURED IN THE UNITED STATES OF AMERICA

S   10   9   8   7   6   5   4   3   2

To our spouses Vera Byers and Fred Goerner—and to all persons who have ever been called hypochondriacs, neurotic, or mentally ill while struggling to cope with their allergies.

Contents

Introduction

Chapter 1 **BREAKTHROUGHS ON THE ALLERGY FRONT** 13
Two Types of Allergy 14
The Changing Patient 25
What Allergy Isn't 27
Tracking Down Your Type 32

Chapter 2 **PORTRAIT OF A TYPE 1** 37
Type 1 Symptoms 38
Type 1 Allergens 42
Testing, Testing 44
New Treatments for Type 1 Persons 48

Chapter 3 **PORTRAIT OF A TYPE 2** 63
Type 2 Symptoms 64
Type 2 Allergens 71
Testing, Testing 77
New Treatments for Type 2 Persons 82
The Universal Reactor 87
The Ecology Unit 89

Chapter 4 **ALL ABOUT FOODS** 95
The Four Food Reactions 96
The Food Sensitivity Diets 99
Challenge Yourself 115
Alcoholism, Obesity, and the 5/5 Allergy-Obesity Diet 118
Cooking Hints 130

Chapter 5   **HELP YOURSELF TO HEALTH**   **135**
Cleaning House   **135**
Allergens at Work   **142**
Tips for Travel   **147**
Choosing a Doctor   **152**

Chapter 6   **ALTERNATIVE TECHNIQUES**   **161**
Mind Techniques   **161**
Body Techniques   **168**

Chapter 7   **WHAT'S IN THE FUTURE**   **177**
Therapies to Come   **178**
Fewer Prescription Drugs   **182**
No More Allergies   **183**

GLOSSARY   **187**

APPENDICES   **193**
1   Biological Food Families   **193**
2   Foods Most and Least Likely to Cause Allergic
Reactions   **201**

WHERE TO SEND FOR PRODUCTS   **203**

REFERENCES   **215**

INDEX   **217**

ACKNOWLEDGMENTS

Very special thanks to Janice Gallagher, friend and editor, for her support, encouragement, and unlimited patience; to Dr. Sandor Burstein, Dr. Phyllis Saifer and Dr. Mark Saifer, Dr. René Bine and Dr. Glenn Nesty; to assistants Marjorie Grannan, Peggy Rolandson, and Jacqueline Young-de Roover; and to Fred Hill, Dev Kettner, Gary Zellerbach, and Lottie and Ed Sugarman for various areas of help along the way.

Note: The word "he" is used in this book as shorthand for "he and she" and is not meant to imply gender discrimination, male superiority, or the authors' laziness.

A man's own observation, what he finds good of, and what he finds hurt of, is the best physic to preserve health.

Francis Bacon, Essays, *VII*, *1597*

INTRODUCTION

This is a book for the mildly allergic; for the severely allergic; for those of you who suspect you might be allergic; and for many who may not realize that your annoying, distressing, or crippling symptoms can be signs of simple or complex allergies. The pages that follow should provide answers to your questions and, if necessary, direct you to the best medical care for your needs.

The field of allergy is one of the fastest-growing areas in medicine and one of the most fruitful spheres of biochemical research. The late 1970s and early 1980s have seen many new discoveries, developments, and refinements, not only in diagnosis and treatment but also in understanding the different physiological mechanisms that cause symptoms, some of which have never before been linked with allergies.

These findings can help you right now. The success of current medical advances depends on you—the person suffering some degree of discomfort or ill health—rather than on drugs, doctors, or hospitals. This is especially true with allergies, because only you can control the amount of exposure you get to allergy-causing substances in your environment.

The chapters that follow will guide you through the steps to help you understand and diagnose your own symptoms, using the latest information. You may find that a few changes of diet or lifestyle are all that is necessary. Or if you feel you need medical care, you'll want to know how to choose the right physician.

Equally important is the realization that your problem may not be an allergy. Both patients and doctors sometimes get caught up in medical fads and rush to attach unnecessary labels. Seemingly allergic symptoms can have other physical or emotional causes that should be ruled out before you seek any kind of specialized treatment.

These pages will provide a much larger and broader picture of allergy than the limited scope of currently available literature. There has never been a time in medical history when so many breakthroughs have occurred in such a short span of years. Yet the general public and most physicians are unaware of the leaps in progress that have recently been made.

We're excited about all the new findings and possibilities, particularly the fact that many years of research have finally culminated in the division of allergy into two main types. The Type 1 category covers the traditional concept of respiratory and skin disorders resulting from specific inhalants such as pollens, dust, animal dander, and molds. Type 2 encompasses a much wider and more complex range of symptoms, mainly attributed to sensitivities to foods and chemicals.

Our purpose in writing this book is to give you all the new options you won't find in any other allergy guide and to put you back in control of your life. With your awareness and your dedicated application of the principles outlined here, we believe you can soon be launched on a safe and steady journey to lasting allergy relief.

Chapter 1

BREAKTHROUGHS ON
THE ALLERGY FRONT

It was early May 1981 when Merla, the patient half of this writing team, first stepped into the office of Al, the medical half. He had been recommended by her family doctor, who thought it might be helpful to try a new approach for controlling allergies—a treatment that didn't depend on drugs.

She was a tough case, having seen allergists since infancy, having tried every conventional medication, yet still struggling with a runny nose, postnasal drip, and chronic laryngitis. On the positive side, she had nothing to lose but her illness—and her skepticism that she would one day recover.

The doctor took a long medical history, asked a few questions she thought odd ("Do you cook on a gas stove? Do you work in a new building?"), and then sent her in to Debbie Dadd, his technician, to be tested for substances to which she might be allergic. The waiting room was crowded, and as the new patient sat down, a man in the next chair began to squirm uncomfortably. He very pointedly took out something that looked like a miniature gas mask and covered his nose.

"Are you all right?" she asked.

"You're wearing deodorant!" he snarled.

Guilty. She admitted it. Was something wrong? Debbie whispered that many people are highly sensitive to aftershave, hairspray, soap, and other perfumed products and that all persons are asked not to use such items before coming to the office. The appointment had been made on brief notice; otherwise, the new patient would have received, in the mail, explicit instructions on how to divest herself of odors. Would she mind moving a few feet away?

Banished to scented seclusion, she had time to scan the printed sheet on testing procedures. She read about the *sublingual* (under the tongue) method, but it still came as a surprise when Debbie squirted some drops of test substances called *antigens* under her tongue; handed her a pencil, a pad, and an egg-timer; and told her to set it for ten minutes and write down any reactions. Luckily there were none.

But a young woman who'd been laughing and joking had taken some drops a moment before. In that short testing interval, she became pale and somber, buried her face in her hands, and began to weep. Debbie dispensed another sublingual squirt and, to everyone's relief, the woman dried her tears, sat very still for five minutes, then opened her eyes, looked up, and smiled. What was going on? Was this the office of a physician or a witch doctor? What kind of drops had the magical power to make a person sad or happy?

Debbie explained that she had been testing for two chemicals, phenol and ethanol, both of which can cause sudden mood changes. Since the new patient showed no response to the chemicals, Debbie proceeded to another technique known as *intradermal*, which involves injecting different antigens into the top layer of skin on the upper arm. The immediate eruption of large itchy wheals left little doubt as to the reaction.

Three days and innumerable tests later, the doctor took the new patient into his office. She wasn't the least surprised to hear that she was sensitive to house dust, grass and tree pollens, cats, dogs, and molds. She wasn't surprised to learn that she had an angry red throat and a badly inflamed nose. She wasn't surprised to hear that she needed immediate attention. She was surprised, however, to hear herself labeled "a typical Type 1." She was soon to learn what that intriguing term meant.

TWO TYPES OF ALLERGY

The designation of Type 1 and Type 2 allergies is unique to this book, but the concept is familiar to the many physicians and researchers who have been pondering these categories in recent years. One day in 1981, when the doctor was discussing a patient with a colleague, he found himself saying that the woman had "traditional allergic symptoms: respiratory inflammation, facial swelling, hand eczema—the first type of reaction, not the second type." Without giving it more thought, he noted in the file that she suffered "classic Type 1 allergic rhinitis." That casual inscription gave birth to a terminology that he and his office staff have been using ever since.

To be specific, a Type 1 person is anyone with "traditional" allergic responses to pollens, dust, animal dander, molds, bee stings, wool and other natural fibers, and some foods. Type 1 patients sneeze, wheeze, cough, scratch, ache, and look puffy, because the primary target organs for Type 1 reactions are the nose and respiratory system, the skin, eyes, ears, gastrointestinal tract, and, occasionally, the brain.

In contrast, a Type 2 person reacts mainly to chemicals in the environment and to foods and their additives. Symptoms vary widely and seem unrelated to conventional notions of allergy. The most surprising and dramatic Type 2 reactions are the cerebral and behavioral responses, which include migraine headaches, confusion, memory loss, personality changes, mood swings, hyperactivity, and depression.

Most Type 1 allergies start at infancy or in childhood and result from an inherited tendency plus exposure to foods, pollens, dust, and other organic substances. Symptoms may subside in early adulthood or continue for a lifetime.

Type 2 allergies usually first appear in hyperactive children or in adults in their twenties or later, and—possibly because of hormonal changes—affect more women than men. Symptoms spring from heavy exposure to chemicals, or a viral illness, and subside when chemicals are avoided.

There is no absolute straight line dividing Type 1 and Type 2 *allergens*—substances that cause allergies—any more than one can say that all people have only Type 1 or Type 2 symptoms. Depending on the weather, other illnesses they may have, emotional stresses, and degree of exposure, the line may blur. A Type 1 hay-fever victim might develop a Type 2 sensitivity to the pesticide sprayed on his crops. A chemically allergic Type 2 might become intolerant of house dust. But even with the occasional overlap, the majority of people fall into one category or the other. Chapters 2 and 3 explain this aspect of allergies in detail.

You might wonder how such different groups of symptoms can be said to be the same ailment. The answer is that both fit the traditional definition of allergy: *adverse responses to substances that don't cause adverse responses in most people.* Both are the result of impaired white blood cells known as *T cells*, which leave the immune system unable to function as it should. And both are governed by your *tolerance threshold.*

To understand the term "tolerance threshold," think of the proverbial straw that broke the camel's back. You can endure a certain amount of exposure to dust or chemicals or whatever you're allergic to without having symptoms. But once you pass a point and cross that threshold, your system has been overloaded with allergens and you react. Every human being, in fact, is allergic; it's just that people who are "not allergic" have never passed their tolerance thresholds.

A glance at the following lists should provide a better idea of the differences in the two types of response. Remember that this is just a guideline; Type 1 persons sometimes get Type 2 symptoms, and Type 2 persons can get every possible symptom known to psychiatry and medicine. Since the range of Type 2 symptoms would fill a chapter in itself, this listing is limited to reactions that seem typical.

The most common Type 1 symptoms occur mainly in response to dust, pollens, animal dander, molds, and foods, and include the following:

RESPIRATORY

Hay fever and asthma
Itchy, teary, red eyes
Swollen lids
Dark circles under eyes (allergic shiners)
Sensitivity to light
Sinus headache
Facial swelling or puffiness
Pain or pressure in ears

Sensitivity to loud sounds
Congested nose, watery discharge, sneezing
Loss of ability to smell or taste
Itching and tingling of mouth and palate
Sore throat from postnasal drip
Loss of voice
Hypersensitivity to heat, cold, temperature changes
Coughing, wheezing, difficulty in breathing
Chest pain

GASTROINTESTINAL

Nausea and vomiting
Abdominal pain or cramps
Diarrhea

GENITOURINARY

Frequent urination
Urgency of urination
Bedwetting

SKIN

Eczema (a dry, itchy rash)
Hives, local or generalized
Angioedema (giant hives associated with swelling)
Itching and redness from insect bites, possible throat swelling and
    shock reaction

SYSTEMIC

Chills
Fatigue

CEREBRAL

Sinus headache
Loss of appetite
Dizzy spells, lightheadedness
Irritation, malaise

The most common Type 2 symptoms occur mainly in response to synthetic chemicals and foods, and include the following:

RESPIRATORY

Dry mouth
Ringing in ears
Sensitivity to odors

GASTROINTESTINAL

Gain in weight
Craving for food, alcohol, or tobacco
Constipation

GENITOURINARY

Chronic bladder irritation
Bedwetting
Premenstrual tension
Menstrual cramps

SKIN

Sweating
Flushing

SYSTEMIC

Fluid retention in any part of body
Unexplained fluctuation of weight
Muscle and joint swelling, redness and pain
Backache
Fatigue

CARDIOVASCULAR

Abnormal heart rhythms
Severe chest pain

CEREBRAL

Migraine headache
Changes of mood: lack of ability to concentrate; feelings of sadness, weariness, frustration, animation, euphoria, aggressiveness, anger, panic, violence, silliness, "spaciness"
Inappropriate laughter
Crying spells
Impairment of speaking and reading ability
Lack of coordination
Loss of balance
Excessive hunger or thirst
Sleepiness or insomnia
Phobias, delusions, hallucinations
Amnesia
Convulsive seizures
Blackouts
Psychosis such as manic depression or schizophrenia

The evolution of the distinction between these two types has been slow and complex, and dates back to 1906 when an Austrian pediatrician named Clemens von Pirquet first coined the word *allergy*—meaning "altered reactivity"—to describe the symptoms of hay fever. The definition gradually came to be "responses to substances that affect some people and not others."

In the 1920s Dr. Albert Rowe made medical history by publishing his well-documented reports of food allergies, closely followed by Dr. Arthur Coca's findings that allergic reactions increased the heartbeat and accelerated the pulse. He formulated a simple but effective *pulse test* (described in Chapter 2) that gave many people insight into their illnesses and helped them isolate their reactions to specific foods.

Although the nomenclature didn't exist at the time, Dr. Coca understood not only both Type 1 and Type 2 reactions to foods but also that the same food might cause a Type 1 person to sneeze or cough and a Type 2 person to feel abnormal tiredness or depression.

Dr. Herbert Rinkel uncovered the mystery of food addiction

in the 1930s, which led to the identification of four different food reactions: *fixed, cumulative, variable,* and *addictive.* They pertain to both Types 1 and 2, and merit a brief explanation.

Some people become nauseated every time they eat peanuts; others feel their lips swell at the first bite of cantaloupe. If you always get the same symptoms from the same food, you're said to have a *fixed* reaction. A *cumulative* reaction means that allergens have to accumulate in your body. You could eat the offending food at several different meals before getting symptoms, which makes it difficult to trace the cause. A *variable* response is unpredictable; bacon may give you hives one morning and a headache the next. Dr. Rinkel's contribution was the discovery that some reactions are *addictive*—that is, you can become addicted to foods the same way you can be hooked on drugs. We'll explain more about these processes in Chapter 4.

To summarize briefly, both Type 1 and Type 2 persons can have all four kinds of food reaction, although addiction is more common with Type 2s. Both can have Type 1 symptoms such as stuffy noses and skin rashes, but Type 1s rarely have Type 2 cerebral symptoms such as sudden, unexplained changes of mood. Both are mainly sensitive to the same foods: milk, wheat, eggs, corn, yeast, soy, citrus fruit, nuts, beef, and some seafood. Both, too, can reduce their food reactions with the now-familiar rotation diet, another of Dr. Rinkel's contributions.

It works this way: you eat one food a meal and wait four days before eating it again, to prevent overloading the system with allergens. The rotation technique was a major step in controlling food sensitivities, and is still widely used today.

The standard rotation diet is based on a division of foods into biological families (see Appendix 1), a system formulated in 1930 by Dr. Warren Vaughan. It classifies foods according to similar appearance and physical structure. If you ate a lemon for lunch, you would wait four days before eating an orange, since they're both members of the same biological food family. The fact that lemons and oranges look alike and have almost identical anatomies is assumed to mean that they cause the same kind of allergic reactions, but this assumption has recently been challenged.

In 1980 Robert W. Gardner, Ph.D., of Brigham Young University in Provo, Utah, introduced his theory that foods with similar structures are not necessarily similar in their biochemical composition and, therefore, are not necessarily similar in their allergens. He suggested that a group of chemical compounds called *phenyls*, contained in foods and other substances, may be the common denominator of allergic reactions.

At this moment there is no reason to believe the phenyl grouping is superior to the biological food families, but Dr. Gardner's work has revealed the possibility that there may be other and better ways to classify foods. His research is still being studied, and evidence indicates that it may be useful in the future.

Dr. Vaughan's biological food families and Dr. Rinkel's rotation diet and food-addiction discoveries were the milestones of the 1930s. The field of allergy again exploded in the late 1940s, with Dr. Theron Randolph's remarkable observation that not only foods but seemingly harmless synthetic chemicals in homes, workplaces, and industrial areas can cause a variety of mental and physical problems, later to be identified as Type 2 responses. Up to this time, there had only been one recognized form of allergy, which we now know as Type 1.

Scratch tests were the prevailing method of diagnosis, and many conventional doctors still think they're the best technique available today. It might be valuable to note the distinction between *allergen* and *antigen*, although for our purposes the words are interchangeable. Both generally refer to foreign substances that come into the body and stimulate the formulation of *antibodies*, tiny molecules that fight them off. "Antigen" is a broader term that includes viruses and bacteria as well as inhalants; an allergen is a specific antigen (pollen, dust, formaldehyde, and so forth) that causes allergies.

In the scratch test, a concentrated extract of allergen is scratched onto the patient's arm or back, penetrating only the outermost layer of skin. The size and redness of the wheal that appears after twenty minutes determines the degree of Type 1— and only Type 1—sensitivity.

If a patient has a positive reaction to a substance such as grass pollen, the doctor then starts him on a series of *desensitizing shots*. He injects a tiny amount of the actual pollen extract and gradually increases the dose over many months until the patient builds up a tolerance. In most cases, the patient can then inhale a reasonable amount of grass pollen without reacting.

The lay public first became aware of a different kind of test with the appearance, in 1979, of Dr. Marshall Mandell's *5-Day Allergy Relief System*. He described a technique called *provocative-neutralization* (P-N), which had been developed by Dr. Carleton Lee in the early 1960s and later modified by Dr. Joseph Miller of Alabama. P-N employs sublingual drops to diagnose Type 2 chemical and other allergies that scratch tests are unable to detect.

The test is called "provocative" because it seeks to provoke an allergic response. First the tester squirts drops of the suspected allergen under the tongue. The skin under the tongue is thinner than that on the arms, back, and buttocks, so the drops are immediately absorbed into the system. The patient counts to 30, then swallows. If there are any symptoms within ten minutes, he records them on a special form.

The great advantage of this method is that first the tester provokes an exact allergic reaction to a suspected substance, and then can usually eliminate these symptoms by giving another sublingual dose of the same substance, only a weaker dilution.

The technique is not voodoo, magic, or imagination. It is based on solid immunological principles that are complex to explain. A specific concentration of antigen will immediately turn off an allergic reaction to that same antigen in approximately 70 percent of Type 1 and Type 2 patients. The relief can last from forty-five minutes to several days; then the extract has to be administered again.

Dr. Mandell's book alerted the public to these somewhat startling innovations as well as to the work of Dr. Theron Randolph and other pioneers in the field. Many scientists and laypersons soon came to the realization that the nose, throat, and skin ailments commonly referred to as allergies are but a fraction of the problem, and that sensitivities to chemicals and pollutants in the environment constitute a vast and challenging part of this same illness.

The study and treatment of this speciality has come to be called *clinical ecology*. The growing group of doctors who practice this environmental approach to allergy use diagnostic and treatment methods that are no different in principle from those used by traditional allergists, but their techniques are expanded, sophisticated, refined, highly personalized, and speeded-up.

Clinical ecologists treat both Type 1 and Type 2 patients with P-N (provocative-neutralization) therapy specific to each type. They have adapted the principles of P-N to a form of skin testing called *intradermal*, which is more sensitive than scratch tests and sometimes provokes Type 1 patients to respond systemically (with a headache, chills, or the like) as well as producing a localized skin wheal. Drugs aren't used in treatment unless absolutely vital.

The medical establishment as a whole has not given its blessing to these new ideas, and certainly the drug industry is underwhelmed; even so, every month two or three scientific studies appear to corroborate and substantiate what clinical ecologists are doing.

Dr. Mandell's disclosure opened a world of possibilities to millions of persons who had erroneously been labeled as neurotic, hysterical, or hopelessly psychotic. The discovery of chemical allergies was a quantum leap in medical history, and scientists continue to make impressive strides. This book will cover the most significant refinements and breakthroughs of the last four years. The biochemical mechanisms of Type 1 and 2 responses, for instance, no longer baffle researchers who look to the body's immune system for the key.

The immune system's job is to process all foreign substances entering the body and render them harmless. Because it works mainly through white blood cells, which travel through every artery and capillary, the immune system spreads to every organ in the body.

There are many kinds of white blood cells; the two involved in immune reactions are *T cells* and *B cells*. T cells direct B cells to produce antibodies—protein molecules that attack foreign substances. Type 1 persons inherit specific allergy-related T cells and overactive B cells from their ancestors. These T cells are unable to do their job—that is, they can't tell the B cells which foreign substances are benign and which are dangerous, so the B cells start producing antibodies indiscriminately. When they overload us with a particular antibody called *IgE* (immunoglobulin E), we get a

Type 1 allergic reaction. The more IgE the B cells produce, the worse we feel.

In contrast, most Type 2 persons are not oversupplied with IgE. Doctors who feel that allergy, by definition, demands a high count of IgE antibodies do not consider Type 2 persons, who usually have a low count, to be truly allergic. Their focus on this difference fails to take into account that both reactions fit the basic definition of allergy, including the fact that both are immune-system malfunctions with T cell deficiencies.

In a Type 2 person, a different kind of B cell produces a different kind of antibody known as *IgG* (immunoglobulin G). An overabundance of IgG linked with an antigen causes Type 2 symptoms, which, as we mentioned, can be anywhere and every where in the body and can range from mild sweating to full-blown psychosis. Some doctors find it hard to accept that exposure to physical substances can cause mental disorders, but this has been proven and documented in literally hundreds of medical texts and papers since 1972.

The major advance in allergy in the last few years has been the realization that the immune system is continuously switched on, like a car with its engine running. The B cells are the car's engine, and the T cells are the brakes. Allergic people, both Types 1 and 2, have high-powered engines (B cells) and weak brakes (T cells), so their car—or immune system—often goes out of control. In other words, an allergic reaction means that you have lost partial control of your immune system. This is a significant new discovery.

Type 1 allergies have been prominent in the past because people have inherited weak brakes (T cells). In Type 2 allergies, the brakes are usually weakened by outside factors synonymous with modern civilization, such as chemicals, stress, and infectious disease. In both types of allergy, immunotherapy readjusts the brakes; that is, it trains the T cells to become stronger and function as they should.

Scientists are seeking new ways to enhance and strengthen these T cells by using either drugs or the body's own materials. Dr. David Katz of La Jolla, California, has isolated a substance from the T cells, injected it into mice, and found that it reduces levels of IgE, the antibody that causes Type 1 symptoms. Dr. Richard Hamburger of San Diego is attempting to take a small section of the IgE molecule and somehow use it as a bogus IgE to fool the body into not reacting. These complicated procedures are still very much in the testing stage.

As you read on, you'll gain a better understanding of the two types of allergy as well as of the "universal reactor" who combines both types and is sensitive to almost everything, but who nevertheless responds well to treatment. By the time you finish this chapter, you should know which tag, if any, to pin on yourself. The advantage of this knowledge is that it can help you to modify your diet and your environment by eliminating certain substances that you may never have guessed were making you ill. It can also help you choose a doctor and decide which kinds of tests and therapies are best for you. Type 2 treatment does little for Type 1 patients and vice versa.

Before you confirm your diagnosis in the next two chapters, let's answer a question that has probably crossed your mind: Why have allergies suddenly become so prominent?

THE CHANGING PATIENT

In the 1950s medical statisticians used to say that one in every seven persons was allergic. In the 1970s the figure jumped to one in five. Today it's estimated that one in every three persons in the United States, or a total of 75 million Americans, has some sort of symptom, minor or major, that can be traced to an allergy.

One reason for this spectacular increase is that many more symptoms are being recognized, identified, and attributed to allergies. The second reason is that *any* substance in the environment can cause a reaction. It can be a flower, a strawberry, your favorite old wool sweater, or fumes from the paint in your new quartz heater. It would not be unusual for you to react to such everyday items as the plastic in your telephone or the exhaust gases from the bus or car that takes you to work.

The third and perhaps most important reason is that the average citizen of the 1980s is biochemically and genetically different from the average citizen of the 1950s. We are so different, in fact, that ordinary medical texts and training are geared to treat people who no longer exist.

It is only during the last twelve years that doctors and scientists have come to realize the immense immune problems we face. The malfunctioning of the immune system commonly known as allergy affects a huge number of people who have been diagnosed as having everything from executive burnout to rheumatoid arthritis. And this number keeps growing.

The current figure of one in three doesn't even include the many persons who show some manifestation of symptoms without suspecting they may have allergies. They're unaware of the possibility because they don't recognize how or why we have so markedly changed. Here are the prime reasons:

1. Our population now includes first- and second-generation descendants of people who would never have survived without antibiotics, insulin, or other modern therapies; thus, the genetic makeup—the actual physiology of the human body—is quite different from what it was only ten or twenty years ago.

2. The birth-control pill and the marked swing in social mores have increased the transmission of viral and parasitic diseases through sexual contact. Also, jet travel has expanded geographic mobility and exposed people to many new foreign bacteria and viruses. The result is that some infectious diseases which were rarely seen in our population five years ago are now widespread.

3. Building and ventilation techniques have changed so drastically for the worse because of energy conservation that it's not unusual for a working person to breathe contaminated air filled with toxins and infectious particles for four to eight hours at a time. This was unheard of even twenty years ago.

4. The vast increase of chemicals in our environment, foods, and medicines has greatly altered the body's ability to rid itself of toxins. The number of untested chemicals used to make everyday products keeps multiplying. Soil, air, and water are polluted with chemical wastes. Even our homes, which have been overinsulated in well-intended attempts to save energy, act as sealed pockets of hazardous fumes.

These factors have changed the character of illness and disease so much that the average physician can no longer rely on past case histories or textbooks but must depend on the immediate observation of the patient.

More than ever before, it's your own responsibility to understand your condition and take deliberate steps to get well. One of the first and most important things you can do is to ascertain that allergy is truly your problem.

WHAT ALLERGY ISN'T

Whether you're a longtime Type 1 sufferer or a newly diagnosed Type 2, you have the same goal: to enhance your body's ability to heal itself and restore inner balance, preferably without the use of drugs. This equilibrium process is called *homeostasis* or, simply, good health.

To achieve this happy state, you need to make sure you've charted the right course. Too many people take false hope from misleading ads and articles that offer instant diagnosis via a *cytotoxic* (blood toxin) test or that promise immediate relief for every known ailment. Such easy bait always contains a hook.

Food reactions, too, can sometimes lead to wrong conclusions. Indigestion or heartburn may be just that. An allergic person is often tempted to attribute all food reactions to allergies, thus depriving himself not only of the pleasure of eating certain dishes but also of their nutrients. Conversely, many people blame their symptoms on other substances or causes when the culprits actually are in their diet. The best way to know which reactions are not food allergies is to sample the suspect items in a home-testing situation that you control yourself. We explain how to do this in Chapter 4.

Allergies are very much in vogue right now, and their trendy status warrants caution. A woman we'll call Nancy is a prime example. In 1982 she was 31 years old, twenty pounds underweight, anemic, and distraught. A year before, she had been having vision problems for which her ophthalmologist had found no cause. A friend recommended she try an ecology center in Southern California. At this small outpatient medical facility,

Nancy was interviewed by a therapist, not an M.D., who didn't examine her physically or listen to what she was saying, but promptly told her, "Your blurred vision is an allergy and we can cure it."

He started her on a strict rotation diet (one that allows foods to be repeated only at four-day intervals), administered sublingual tests, and gave her antigens (drops) to take every six hours. When Nancy began to feel worse and lose weight, her requests to see the doctor on the staff went unheeded. She soon became so run down that she started getting symptoms from foods she had never reacted to before.

"It was a horrendous experience," she recalls. "I knew I had to go off that diet even though the clinic staff frightened me and told me I would have terrible problems if I did."

She finally stopped the diet and the drops, and she did have bad symptoms for several months. Now, a year later, she has gained back fifteen of her twenty pounds, solved her eye problems by wearing glasses instead of contact lenses, and is just beginning to feel healthy again. "The fault was mine," she admits. "I should have checked out the ecology center with my doctor. Had I known I wasn't going to be treated by an M.D., I never would have gone."

There is a moral to this story: Don't rush to the nearest "ecology center" without knowing exactly what kind of facility it is, what kind of medical supervision it has, and whether you truly are a candidate for that type of care.

Chances are that you're not. The average allergic person doesn't need drastic measures. Unless your symptoms are severe and disabling, you would be wiser to focus your efforts on learning exactly what your allergies are (if, indeed, you do have them) and then working to eliminate the offenders that surround you. Be sure that any physician who treats you for allergy takes a thorough medical history, examines you physically, and tests you in controlled conditions before making a diagnosis.

The following checklist will help you rule out some common body symptoms that should *not* be treated as allergies. This will prevent you from taking a wrong direction in seeking relief and from wasting time that might cost dearly if you're suffering a different type of disorder.

From Head to Toe:
An Allergy-or-Not Checklist

YES—*this probably is an allergic symptom*

NO—*this probably is not an allergic symptom*

HEAD

Migraine headache

A headache that's worse when you awaken in the morning but rapidly improves when you sit upright

Sinus headache

A headache associated with stiff neck and fever

Muscle-tension headache, especially after eating the wrong food

A headache associated with loss of muscle control, especially in anal sphincter or bladder

EYES

Blurred vision associated with eating certain foods or smelling certain odors
Visual changes associated with specific geographic locations

Double vision when looking hard to the right or left

Loss of vision in one or both eyes
Unequal size of the pupils
Yellowness in the eyeballs
Pain or swelling in one eye only
Rapid deterioration of vision

EARS

Ringing or buzzing
Recurrent infections
Blocked
Itching
Sounds too loud or very soft
Intermittent hearing losses

Pain in one ear only
Infection accompanied by fever, pain, and swelling below or behind the ear
Deafness, vertigo, nausea, and a tendency to fall in one direction

NOSE

A thin, clear discharge

Recurrent nosebleeds

Sneezing fits
Itchy nose and palate

A thick, yellowish-green discharge
Severe nosebleed with high blood pressure

MOUTH AND THROAT

Difficulty swallowing
Chronic sore throat with no known causes
Chronic dry feeling

Chemical taste in the mouth
Sudden change of voice

A painless lump in the throat
Sore throat associated with fever

Persistent cough without fever in smokers
Chronic sore on the tongue
Gradual change in voice

NECK

Stiff neck not associated with injury or trauma
Thyroid malfunction

Stiff neck associated with fever
Painful lymph glands down front or back of the neck
Bulging neck veins, which become worse when you are lying down

CHEST

Wheezing
Severe chest pain
Irregular heartbeat

Recurrent pneumonia episodes

Wheezing from one lung only
Chest pain associated with fever
Chest pain associated with sweating, clammy skin, and fainting
Shortness of breath associated with nausea and/or heart palpitations
Labored breathing that is worse when you are lying flat, and

is associated with swollen
ankles or belly

BREASTS

Equal swelling

Swelling or lump on one side
only
Black or yellowish discharge
from the nipples

ABDOMEN

Chronic or temporary diarrhea
Bloating after meals

Blood in stool
Pain that starts below the
breastbone and radiates to the
back
Severe pain with or without
fever
Pain that starts below the
breastbone and radiates to the
right of the rib cage
Pain that starts at the navel and
descends to the right lower
quadrant of the belly

BACK

Aching associated with other
muscle and joint aches

Pain that radiates down to the
vulva or testes
Pain associated with fever

GENITOURINARY

Bedwetting
Frequent or urgent urination

Recurrent vaginal yeast infections

Blood or pus in urine
Frequent or urgent urination
with fever
Skin eruptions on the penis or
vulva

Loss of libido

Loss of stool or urine without the sensation of passing stool or urine

LIMBS

Pain in joints and/or muscles

Fatigue that feels as if limbs are made of lead

Hands turn blue in cold water

Sudden loss of control of one or more limbs

Swelling of lower limbs associated with shortness of breath, especially at night

SKIN

Red, itchy rash

Rash weeping yellow discharge or pus

CEREBRAL

Behavioral changes with no obvious reason
Job burnout
Hyperactivity
Unexplained depression

Emotional reaction to a trauma

To summarize, call a doctor immediately in any instance of severe pain or bleeding, high fever, or sudden body irregularities. Most of these symptoms could be allergies, although many are not.

Now that you know the pitfalls of labeling every sneeze, ache, or itch an allergy, you'll want to know more about the common and uncommon symptoms that do fit the definition.

TRACKING DOWN YOUR TYPE

There is something important you should know about yourself before you go any further: Are you a Type 1, a Type 2, a combination of both, or a universal reactor? You may not need the services of an allergist to find out. Understanding your type may answer a lot of puzzling questions and help you to solve your own health problems. If you do decide to see a specialist, however, you'll be able to supply information that will save time and money in the diagnostic process.

This quiz will tell you what you want to know. We've divided it into three parts so that you can determine whether your symptoms are caused mainly by factors in the environment, by foods, or by food addiction. Take your time and think about each answer. You may have to do some research on yourself before completing the tests.

Part 1: Environment

On a separate sheet of paper, write down the number—0, 1, or 2—that best expresses your reaction to each environment. If necessary, test yourself in the actual situations. Compare how you feel breathing fresh air at the seashore and how you feel at some of the places listed. Become hyperattuned to yourself. If you think you already know how you react, then you can complete the test now.

KEY

0—No reaction
1—Any of the following: congested or runny nose, sneezing, mouth and palate tingle, sore throat, difficulty with breathing, chills, itchy skin or hives, sensations in eyes or ears, stomach cramps, nausea, gas, feeling dizzy or light-headed.
2—Any of the following: sudden mood change expressed by anger, depression, confusion, panic, feeling spacey or elated; hypersensitivity to sounds and odors; bloating and stomach pains; excessive thirst or hunger; any strong craving; headache, muscle or joint aches; palpitations, fatigue; or onset of any other unusual symptoms

A. The detergent section of the supermarket
B. The perfume counter of a department store
C. A florist shop or nursery
D. A candy store
E. A gas station

F. An attic filled with old treasures
G. An office with the newest equipment
H. A pet shop
I. A bus or train station
J. A commercial airliner in flight
K. Your own bedroom
L. An unswept barn or basement
M. A cool, drafty room
N. A traffic jam
O. A room filled with cigarette smoke
P. A picnic on the grass
Q. An area where pesticides have recently been sprayed
R. A seafood restaurant
S. An antique shop or old museum
T. A new energy-sealed office building

Now add up the numbers. If your total score is over 1 and under 10, you're probably a Type 1. If it's over 10 and under 20, chances are you're a Type 2 or a combination of both. If it's over 20, you're extremely allergic and may be a universal reactor.

Part 2: Foods and Beverages

See if this food and beverage test gives you similar results. The key is the same. As before, write down the number—0, 1, or 2—that best expresses your reaction to each item.

A. Apples
B. Beef
C. Bourbon
D. Cantaloupe
E. Cheese
F. Chocolate
G. Coffee
H. Corn
I. Eggs

J. Fish
K. Foods that contain dyes or preservatives
L. Foods with pesticides
M. Milk and milk products
N. Oranges
O. Peanuts
P. Pork
Q. Potatoes
R. Poultry
S. Scotch
T. Shrimp
U. Soy
V. Strawberries
W. Tomatoes
X. Wheat
Y. Wine
Z. Yeast

Score Part 2 separately from Part 1. How many times did you write down the number 2 for the Foods and Beverages test? If you wrote it more than once, you are probably a Type 2 with diet problems that need immediate attention. If you marked the number 1 more than once, you're most likely a Type 1. Even if all your answers were 0, you could still be food-sensitive. Your particular food offender may not be on this list, your reaction might be delayed, or there's a third possibility.

Part 3: Food Addiction

Answer yes or no to these questions:

1. Do you ever feel a strong craving for a particular food?
2. Do you ever feel desperate—that you would go anywhere and pay any price for that food?
3. Do you feel extremely weak, irritable, and frustrated until you satisfy the craving?

4. Do your symptoms disappear when you eat the food?
5. Do you wonder why you can eat and eat and not feel full?

If you answered yes to two or more questions, you're probably a Type 2, addicted to certain foods. You experience similar kinds of withdrawal symptoms when you can't get those foods. This is a common phenomenon and one that can be reversed with willpower and patience. It will be explained in detail in Chapter 4 on food allergies.

The next two chapters will help you discover your type and make clear why a different approach to treatment is necessary for each category. You will read about the most recent testing methods, why some work and some don't, and the newest ways to build up the immune system. Medical therapies require guidance or supervision, so you'll also learn the differences in doctors and their techniques; then you'll be able to choose the approach that suits you best.

The Food Sensitivity Diets provide a way to break bad eating habits, cleanse your body of chemicals it doesn't need, and test yourself for food sensitivities. If your problem is overweight, the 5/5 Allergy-Obesity Diet offers an easy new formula for shedding pounds. A separate chapter explains the best ways to clean up your home and office environments, and also gives suggestions to ease the hidden hazards of travel.

The last two chapters describe alternative treatments for allergies and bring you up to date on the state-of-the-art of medical research and what lies ahead. It should be a bright and healthy future.

Chapter 2

PORTRAIT OF A TYPE 1

The nonmedical author of this book was a colicky infant, full of abdominal cramps and eczema. At two weeks she hadn't the slightest idea that she was starting a typical Type 1 pattern of allergic behavior. Neither did her parents. But she was. Her roster of symptoms included a runny, stuffy nose, coughing, and itchy skin rashes.

At the age of 6 or 7 she suffered a full-blown asthma attack that gradually subsided, only to recur sporadically in those early years. Desensitizing shots helped through the teens, but marriage to a husband who loved boating on pollen-laden rivers and spending summers in the country made for new problems. When they remodeled an old home and moved in before repairs were finished, the moldy wallpaper, dust, and paint fumes were equally disastrous to her nose and throat.

Major surgery some years later intensified the allergies. Her body suddenly seemed "hyperattuned" to all offending substances. She had only to step into a home where a dog or cat resided, for instance, and—even if the animal weren't there or she didn't know the people had a pet—she would react to its airborne dander within minutes. Cold sensitivity became acute, too. Eating an ice cream cone or sipping a chilled drink triggered a sneezing fit. Continuous nasal drip caused a chronic sore throat. All these symptoms became worse when she ate chocolate, eggs, or shellfish. Relief, however, was on the way.

The patient's introduction to clinical ecology in 1981 was both startling and educational. At first she was confused by the new ways of testing and treatment, but gradually she began to learn the difference between the two types of allergy and why her particular group of symptoms merited a particular kind of therapy.

One hesitates to use the word "cured" in respect to allergy, but she feels very fortunate that environmental changes and medical care relieved her major symptoms, freed her of a dependence on antihistamines, and lifted the heavy allergic burden she had carried for so many years. If you think you may be a Type 1 person, check out the road signs ahead.

TYPE 1 SYMPTOMS

Allergic Rhinitis: Hay Fever

When the average person thinks of allergy, he thinks of sniffles and runny noses, and with reason. Allergic rhinitis—nasal congestion due to allergies—plagues approximately 22 million Americans, or 10 percent of the population. That's the latest estimate from Dr. Doris J. Rapp, author of *Allergies and Your Family,* and it indicates that this malady is near-epidemic.

Allergic rhinitis is a year-round problem due mainly to airborne inhalants such as house dust, molds, and animal dander. Hay fever is a seasonal ailment due mainly to flower, tree, and plant pollens. Both are the same allergy with typical symptoms of sneezing, watery nasal discharge, itchy palate, postnasal drip, occasional coughing, wheezing, laryngitis, and red, teary eyes.

Sinus headaches often appear when allergic rhinitis causes the nasal passages to swell. Congestion blocks the sinuses so that mucus becomes trapped and can't drain. The result is a dull, persistent pressure above or below the eyes, often on one side only.

A big reason for the increased number of hay fever sufferers is that many of the new chemicals and pollutants in the air add stresses to the body. The pollens, molds, and animal danders that you've lived with for years and that have never bothered you may suddenly combine with atmospheric toxins to push you over your tolerance threshold and cause any or all of the aforementioned symptoms.

Asthma

Most doctors seem to agree that untreated or severe allergic rhinitis can lead to a familiar and sometimes disabling complication. When the bronchial tubes constrict and produce sticky mucus or phlegm, the result is a condition called asthma. Mucus stops up the tubes and obstructs the air flow out of the lungs. When the air tries to squeeze through the narrowed tubes, it makes the sound of wheezing.

An asthma attack can follow a bad cold or bronchitis, but it is mainly an allergic disease. It affects more boys than girls until puberty, when it evens out; more children than adults; more city than country dwellers; and, according to the National Center of Health Statistics, over 10 million Americans.

For many years doctors thought, and some still think, that asthma was a psychosomatic illness caused by emotional problems or stress. Clinical ecologists feel that asthma can be provoked or intensified by stress, but is *caused* by an allergen. If that allergen weren't around there would be no asthma attacks, no matter how great the emotional trauma.

Patients with Type 1 asthma often have a history of infant eczema, hay fever, and sensitivity to foods, pollen, mold spores, animal dander, and dust, as well as having at least one allergic parent. Both hot and cold weather, along with sudden changes in temperature, can aggravate symptoms. Current evidence suggests that this conventional list of causative agents is far too limited, and that asthma can result from food and food additives as well as from exposure to airborne pollutants.

Hormonal changes, such as those produced by menstruation, can also provoke an attack. Dr. Lewis B. Clayton of the American Lung Association theorizes that fluid buildup in a woman's body causes the air passages to swell, making breathing difficult. He suggests that women reduce their salt intake before and during their periods to keep swelling at a minimum.

Smoking, too, is extremely deleterious to asthmatics, and no matter what the Tobacco Institute says, so are secondhand fumes from other people's cigarettes. A 1982 Harvard School of Public Health study found that mothers who smoke "sharply increase" the chances that their children will have asthma and other respiratory illnesses.

Asthma is predominantly a Type 1 symptom but, as you know by now, Type 2 persons can get all Type 1 symptoms (though the reverse is not true), and sometimes they develop severe cases of this illness.

Skin Disorders

The skin is a major target organ for Type 1 allergies, and the main reactions are eczema, hives, and insect-sting responses. Poison ivy and poison oak are included here, but they are not limited to Type 1 persons; Type 2s can be equally susceptible.

Poison ivy and poison oak are different plants from the same family. They are the most common contactants (substances you touch) because their toxicity is so widespread, affecting at least half the population. Those bright "leaves of three" (ivy) and vibrant green and red leaves (oak) are beautiful—but beware. The villain is an oily substance called *urushiol* found in the crushed leaves and stems, not the pollen.

Urushiol is so potent it can be transmitted by a dog or cat who brushes against the plant. It can float on a body of water and infect your skin when you swim. Smoke from burned twigs and leaves can carry it to your face. If only a square inch of your sleeve touches the vine and you put the garment away in a drawer without washing it, you can still get poison ivy or oak from the contaminated spot a year later. Treated or untreated, the rash usually heals by itself in two weeks.

Eczema is specifically a Type 1 skin rash, sometimes called the disease that starts from scratch. It is dry, extremely itchy, and rarely fatal, but it can be unattractive, uncomfortable, and lead to serious skin lesions.

The agents that cause eczema can be any number of contactants, such as perfume, cosmetics, household cleaners, wool or synthetic fabrics, metal, rubber, animal hair or saliva, newsprint, or the skin of such foods as papaya, kiwi fruit, and potatoes. It can be the usual inhalants—dust, pollens, molds, and animal dander—or the fumes of foods or chemicals. Antihistamines are a common cause, as are such drugs as aspirin, penicillin, and hormones. Stress and emotion play a part, but more in aggravating the symptoms than in causing them.

In recent years, progress has been made in tracing eczema to previously unsuspected substances. Cow's milk is still the prime cause in babies, but the rash can also be brought on by indoor and outdoor air pollution, exercise, and extremes of temperature.

Type 1 patients with eczema are advised to avoid close contact with people who have chicken pox or herpes simplex infections. The eczema patient has an immune-system deficiency that makes his skin very vulnerable. If he contracts herpes or chicken pox, he will get a more severe case with possible complications. Also, people with eczema carry more of the bacteria *Staphylococcus aureus* on their skin, so that small lacerations become easily infected and may require treatment with antibiotics.

In contrast to the characteristic red rash of eczema, hives are small, itchy bumps. Their formal name is *urticaria*, and they occur more often in adults than in children, in more females than in males, and, according to Dr. Harsha V. Dehejia, author of *The Allergy Book*, affect as much as 20 percent of the population.

When hives are accompanied by swelling of various parts of the body, especially the mouth, the condition is called angioedema. In severe cases, it can reach the larynx (or voice box), close the breathing pathways, and require an emergency tracheotomy. In general, however, hives are more bothersome than harmful.

Recurrent attacks often appear for no obvious or traceable reason, yet some known causes are foods and food additives, insect bites, intestinal parasites, and exercise. Drugs—mainly aspirin, sulfa and its derivatives, codeine, barbiturates, penicillin (or milk and beef that contain penicillin fed to the cows)—are all common offenders. Sunlight and hot and cold temperatures can cause hives to erupt, as can an emotional trauma such as fear. Some students always break out at exam time.

In general, the causes of hives are broader and may be harder to track down than the causes of eczema. Chronic cases sometimes indicate a more serious disorder such as hepatitis, leukemia, or systemic lupus erythematosus.

The last Type 1 skin disorder is the raised welt that comes from insect bites and stings. Again, although this is a Type 1 response, Type 2 persons can have similar reactions. Stings and bites can usually be distinguished from hives by a tiny hole in the center of the welt. Minor swelling and itching do not constitute an allergy, but abnormal swelling and itching, along with whole-body symptoms such as fever, nausea, hives, difficulty in breathing, or fainting, are definite signs of insect allergy.

Other Type 1 Symptoms

Stomach cramps, nausea, vomiting, heartburn, indigestion, and diarrhea are all gastrointestinal responses that are typically related to foods. These reactions can be either immediate or delayed.

The final Type 1 symptoms that should be mentioned are the cerebral. Hay fever and asthma patients often feel giddy and light-headed, get headaches, or become grouchy and irritable in addition to having skin or respiratory problems. These may be physiological reactions caused by altered brain chemistry, or they may be psychologically induced by the physical discomfort and frustration.

Type 1 symptoms cover the range of responses from the relatively nonthreatening seasonal hay fever to the possibly fatal combination of asthma, hives, and an insect-sting reaction. As you grow older, some of your symptoms may go away by themselves. You'll be able to speed their departure once you know exactly what provokes them.

TYPE 1 ALLERGENS

Any substance that causes symptoms is said to be an allergen. The most common Type 1 allergens are the inhalants: house dust and house dust mites, molds, animal dander (especially from cats and dogs), and tree, weed, and grass pollens. The list also includes foods, mainly milk, wheat, eggs, corn, and yeast.

A Type 1 person can get hay fever or asthma from simply handling mushrooms in the fall, when the fungi are releasing millions of spores and saturating the air with tiny molds. Paradoxically, the person can eat cooked mushrooms with impunity. Some foods, such as egg white, seem to cause the body to release histamine, and are said to be inherently allergenic. In most cases, however, the foods are not exceptionally allergenic in themselves, but cause problems because they are the most commonly eaten, and frequent exposure develops sensitivity.

Various additives can be harmful, too. One common offender is tartrazine, the yellow food dye found in lemon puddings and gelatins, cake mixes, orange- and lime-flavored drinks, beers and liqueurs, processed cheese and "cheese foods," and many pills and vitamins. Tartrazine has no value except to deceive the eye, but it often causes drippy noses, hives, eczema, and asthma in allergy-prone people. Be especially wary of colored dairy products. Several years ago the dairy industry successfully lobbied to avoid having to label its products—to its advantage but to the public's great disadvantage.

The list of Type 1 allergens includes contactants such as aftershave or lipstick; natural fibers in the form of wool, feathers, and goose down; tobacco; drugs and medicines; insect venoms; and cold and heat. All should be familiar except, perhaps, the last two, which merit an explanation.

Cold and heat can act as allergens in three ways: they can be allergens themselves; they can change substances into allergens; and they can intensify existing allergies.

In the first instance, cold serves as a contactant. Some people are so sensitive that their fingers swell when they touch an ice cube. Others erupt in hives from the chilly water of the ocean or swimming pools. Still others must keep themselves bundled up in gloves, earmuffs, and long underwear even in 60-degree weather. If even one small patch of body skin becomes exposed, say a spot of arm or leg, the "leak" will cause symptoms until it's patched. The person who wears three sweaters and an overcoat in a mild climate or who shivers under a blanket when the car window lets in a light breeze is probably a typical Type 1 cold-allergy sufferer.

The second way cold causes symptoms is when lower temperatures produce changes in certain substances, making them more allergenic. One woman couldn't understand why she could drink orange juice at home with no problems, but if she drank it anywhere else she'd start sneezing and coughing. She soon realized that she squeezed fresh, nonrefrigerated oranges at home, but when she drank orange juice in a bar or restaurant it was always chilled. Since other iced drinks didn't bother her, she had to assume that the chilling and perhaps freezing of the orange juice altered some ingredient in it. A good guess is that cold temperatures alter the cell wall structure, breaking down sugar cells so they are more available to the yeast that is often present in orange juice. The yeast would then grow more rapidly and be a more potent allergen.

Third, cold can trigger or aggravate existing allergies. Some Type 1 persons have such sensitive inner thermostats that they respond to a temperature change of even two or three degrees. That slight variation can become an added stress and push them over their tolerance level.

Heat acts in similar ways. As an allergen, it can cause hives and skin rashes. It can change substances by vaporizing solids into harmful gases or by stimulating inert plants to release their pollens. And it can intensify symptoms, because hot air is usually stagnant and holds a higher concentration of dust, molds, and pollens. Warm air can also dry up mucus secretions and plug already obstructed air passages, causing an attack of asthma.

Cold and heat deserve a prominent place on the list of Type 1 allergens, and, for many people, may explain some puzzling symptoms.

TESTING, TESTING

There is a series of tests to identify the allergens causing Type 1 symptoms. They can be done in the office, the laboratory, or the home. In terms of efficiency, skin tests give the most reliable results for inhalant allergens, and challenge testing (done at home) works best for foods and contactants. At present, lab tests have limited use. Let's look first at some of the office procedures.

Office Testing

1. *The Scratch Test.* The tester puts a drop of antigen (a dilution of the test substance) on the skin of the arm or back and then scratches the surface with a needle, allowing the antigen to react with antibodies in the patient's system. If the antibody IgE is present, the wheal will swell and itch, showing a positive reaction. This gives a good indication of Type 1 responses to dust, pollens, animal dander, molds, some drugs such as penicillin, and insect stings. It is not an accurate indication of food allergies, except when there is an immediate severe reaction. At present, scratch tests measure only skin reaction and do not reveal stomach, nose, cerebral, or delayed responses.

2. *The Intradermal Test.* The technician injects a bit of antigen into the skin just beneath the top layer, waits about twenty minutes, and then looks for redness, swelling, and itching—a positive sign. The intradermal is more sensitive and usually gives better results than the scratch test. In a conventional allergist's office, the diagnosis stops there.

3. *The Provocative-Neutralization (P-N) Intradermal Test*. In a clinical ecologist's office, the technician injects a small amount of antigen into the skin, immediately measures the size of the wheal, waits ten minutes, and then measures again to see how much it has grown. The patient records on a sheet of paper any generalized symptoms he may be feeling, such as chills, nasal congestion, or a headache.

The technician continues testing until the correct neutralizing dose is determined from the decreased size of the skin wheal and the cessation of other symptoms. When the specific concentration of antigen that stops the reaction is established, the office part of the test is over. The patient then takes home a diagram of his arm and the test sites, and records any noticeable reactions twenty-four to forty-eight hours later. These responses help the technician to fine tune the dose of antigens.

P-N is not a new procedure but a thoroughly researched refinement of conventional techniques for both testing and treatment. The P-N intradermal test is useful mainly for Type 1 allergies, while the P-N sublingual test determines Type 2 chemical responses and will be described in the next chapter.

Lab Testing

1. *The RAST, or radioallergosorbent test*. This test involves taking a blood sample and measuring the amount of IgE antibodies that form when the blood is exposed to different allergens. The assumption is that the higher the count of IgE antibodies, the more allergic the patient is. The RAST can be moderately useful in diagnosing Type 1 allergies to dust, pollens, molds, animal danders, insect venoms, and some foods. But it has disadvantages, including the following:

It measures only immediate responses, and many allergic reactions are delayed.

It tests for only a limited number of allergens.

It costs two to six times more than skin tests for each allergen tested.

Skin test results are available in 20 to 45 minutes, RAST takes two to three days.

Interpretations and techniques vary; the same blood sent to five different labs may bring five different results.

It can be falsely negative; highly allergic people may show up as "not reactive" on the RAST.

It can be falsely positive; some people with IgE antibodies in their blood do not get allergic symptoms. The mere presence of IgE antibodies is not always proof that the person has become sensitized to the test substance.

On the plus side, the RAST can be useful for infants, who are difficult to test in the office, and for people who have severe rashes or might have dangerous reactions to skin testing. When used in conjunction with other tests it can sometimes confirm a tentative diagnosis.

2. *The Arest Program.* The Iatric Corporation of Tempe, Arizona, has produced a modification of the RAST called the Arest program. It uses radioactive atoms to determine the number of antibodies that respond to a specific allergen, and claims to be able to provide sufficient information to make both a diagnosis and a vaccine for desensitization.

Developers of this new blood test say it is as reliable as the scratch method for Type 1 food and inhalant allergies and will be especially valuable in rural areas and small communities where allergists and specialized treatment are not available. It seems likely, however, that this method will prove to be only slightly better than the RAST.

3. *The Allergy Smear.* In this test, blood, urine, stool, eye, ear, nose, or bronchial secretions are microscopically examined for *eosinophils*, special white blood cells whose presence in large numbers indicates Type 1 allergy. In case of infection or other illness, there would be very few eosinophils. The test is useful when there is some question of diagnosis, but it doesn't pinpoint specific allergens.

4. *The Cytotoxic Test.* This is a widely touted and vastly overrated technique that purports to determine food allergies from a blood sample; more will be said about this in Chapter 3.

Home Testing

1. *The Challenge Test.* This is so-named because you challenge yourself by touching, eating, or inhaling the suspected substance and watching for a reaction. Here are the basic principles of challenge testing:

> Choose any substance you suspect may be giving you symptoms, such as chocolate, wool, or perfume, or choose up to three substances if they're different—one food, one contactant, one inhalant.
>
> Eliminate the test substance 100 percent from your diet or environment for seven days.
>
> At the end of one week, reintroduce a small amount of the substance and see if you get symptoms. This should give you some idea of whether or not you're allergic to it.

Once in a rare while, a doctor will do challenge testing in the office. He'll have you inhale tobacco fumes, apply a cosmetic, or take a few sips of red wine to see what happens. Most doctors, however, have neither the time nor the raw materials for such procedures.

A big advantage of challenge testing is that it can overcome your skepticism. If you insist you can drink brandy, own a dog, or cut the lawn without getting symptoms, for example, you can prove or disprove this yourself. Witnessing your own responses can be a convincing argument to start a diet, give away a pet, or make some other "sacrifice" you have been reluctant to do. Also, taking this step before you consult an allergist will sometimes make medical treatment unnecessary.

Challenge is the most economical way of testing, but it is often cumbersome and can be potentially dangerous. It can be useful for food allergies as long as you follow instructions (see Chapter 4), but if you're sensitive to pollens or respond with severe symptoms such as asthma or bothersome rashes, you had better stick to carefully controlled office testing.

Other disadvantages are that only a few tests can be done at a time, particularly if they evoke strong reactions. Testing may add psychological stress to your tolerance load, and challenging can't be done blind—that is, eliminating effects that result from your expectations. If you're both tester and testee, you can't fool yourself with a placebo.

2. *The Pulse Test.* This technique points you in the direction of your allergies without being overly precise. It was developed by Dr. Arthur Coca in 1956 to detect Type 1 food and inhalant allergies, but today many Type 2 persons use it as well.

Start by checking your pulse rate every two hours to establish your normal range. "Normal" is anywhere from the mid-50s, for physically active people, to the mid-80s, for the less active. The pulse rate fluctuates with every physiological or emotional stress, so daylong monitoring is necessary to get an average.

You can even simplify pulse-taking with a new gadget called the Pulse Tach Fingertip Heart Computer, a microcomputer that weighs one ounce and fits over your fingertip. It's available at $49.95 from Baystar, 100 Painters Mill Road, Dept. 34-T, Owings Mills, MD 21117.

The next step is to take your pulse before introducing a potential allergen, such as a small quantity of rice. Then take your pulse again in five minutes, half an hour, and an hour after you've eaten. A variation of ten or more beats is a sign that you may be allergic to that food. This is based on the principle that an allergic reaction causes the release of adrenalin, which quickens heart and pulse beat. For instance, if your pulse is 63 before consuming rice and half an hour later it's 80, you have good reason to suspect rice.

There are several disadvantages to this test: a stressful phone call or any intrusion will affect the pulse beat; allergens other than the one you're testing may be raising the count; and since you can't test blind, your own expectations can send your pulse soaring. But as allergy tests go, it's simple, safe, and easy on the pocketbook.

NEW TREATMENTS
FOR TYPE 1 PERSONS

Conventional treatment for Type 1 allergies has changed little in the past decade. The first recommendation is still avoidance, followed by medication such as antihistamines and steroids to be taken along with immunotherapy in the form of desensitizing shots.

Clinical ecology treatment is essentially the same. It simply aims to speed those processes and cut down or eliminate the use of drugs. We'll explain some of the newest, the best, and even the worst of both approaches.

For Allergic Rhinitis: Hay Fever

Until very recently, little besides shots, sprays, steroids, and antihistamines has been available to stop the sneezing, coughing, watery eyes, itching, and other familiar trademarks of year-round allergic rhinitis and seasonal hay fever.

Addiction to prescription and nonprescription medication is a staggering problem in the United States, and for this reason clinical ecologists feel that chemotherapy—drug treatment—should be a final resort.

What will replace it? For the last ten years or so, many Type 1 patients have been substituting sublingual antigens with good results. The drops work this way: in your clinical ecologist's office (conventional allergists don't provide this treatment), you undergo several days of P-N intradermal testing. The technician, you will recall, injects a small amount of antigen into your skin and continues this process until the dose that clears your symptoms is determined.

On the final day of testing, the technician gives you one or several bottles containing specific concentrations of extract of the substances to which you're allergic. You take these home and squirt a carefully measured dose, usually three drops, under your tongue once a week, once a day, or up to four times a day if needed. The logical question is whether this technique works in actual life as well as in the office. Can you really turn off an acute Type 1 reaction to house dust by taking a few drops of antigen?

The answer is a scientific yes and a practical maybe. The "maybe" is fourfold:

1. You must have the antigen in the correct neutralizing dilution with you at the time of your reaction. Readjusting the dosage by office testing may often be necessary, especially during pollen season or when you have a virus infection or other sickness.

2. You must ingest exactly the right amount. An extra half drop could make your symptoms worse instead of better.

3. You must be able to pinpoint the offending allergen and take the corresponding antigen. If you take pollen extract when the cat hairs on your friend's sweater are making you sneeze, you won't be helped. If the problem is house dust, you may need to have autogenous dust—that is, dust taken from the vacuum cleaner in your home. This "personalized extract" contains the exact substances you're breathing and is often effective when regular dust antigen is not. It is prepared in a laboratory at the request of your allergist, and is useful if you live in either a very old or very new home or in any area where the dust composition may be unique.

4. You should be able to get away from the allergen so that you are no longer heavily exposed.

If all these factors are right, you may be able to relieve your symptoms immediately and continue in this state until your body builds up a tolerance to the allergens and you no longer need treatment. This is exactly the same principle as desensitizing shots. The main difference is that while you are strengthening your immunity, you may have the means to reduce symptoms naturally rather than having to depend on antihistamines and steroids.

Sublingual drops are effective as desensitizers—that is, for building up immunity in 75 percent of Type 1 patients—but, for the reasons outlined, such as timing or incorrect dosage, they're less successful as neutralizers or immediate symptom relievers.

Clinical ecologists often give shots, or teach patients to inject themselves, when sublingual methods prove ineffective. The same neutralizing doses of antigen (rather than the gradual buildup) can usually effect desensitization in less time than the conventional method.

Two modifications of traditional desensitization treatment have appeared recently. One, called Rush Therapy, works this way: instead of giving the patient two shots a week the first few months and then slowly increasing the strength of the injections, the patient starts out by getting five to eight shots a week in an attempt to speed the rebuilding of the immune system. You might call it a cram course for T cells.

While it seems to be effective for some patients who can tolerate the onslaught of antigens, others get strong allergic reactions and may even go into anaphylactic shock—a very severe allergic reaction characterized by swelling and spasm of the throat tissues, a gasping for breath, and sometimes suffocation and death. There is no way to predict who will be able to tolerate Rush Therapy and who won't.

The second innovation is Allpyral (alum-precipitated-allergen) shots, which incorporate the same principle of immunotherapy, or building up your immune system. The difference is that these injections feed antigen from an alum-based suspension into your system at specific intervals. It's as if you have a time-release capsule in your arm, but instead of getting two shots a week, you get one shot every four weeks. The drawback is that if the dose is wrong, you feel worse for a whole month.

For Asthma

Both conventional doctors and clinical ecologists treat most Type 1 asthmatic patients with injection therapy. Again, the only difference is in dosage and frequency of shots. The principle of building up T cells is the same, but the clinical ecologist tries to do it faster and without accompanying drugs.

Traditional allergists often prescribe steroids for asthma patients. These are powerful hormone compounds that should be used with extreme caution and only in severe cases. Cortisone and prednisone, for example, can cause such serious side effects as high blood pressure, brittle bones, kidney problems, weight gain and bloating, and even cataracts and diabetes. They can also inhibit the action of the adrenal glands to produce their own cortisone in times of stress, thus lowering the body's resistance to bacterial, fungal, and viral infections.

As with all allergy drugs now on the market, steroids treat symptoms, not the cause, by turning off certain parts of the immune system so that the body doesn't react to allergens. At the same time, they also turn off the body's defenses against disease. It must be said, however, that cortisone in its various forms has helped many more people than it has harmed.

Cromolyn sodium (brand name: Intal) is another widely used

medication. Many asthmatics find that if they inhale this white powder fifteen minutes before exercising, it inhibits spasms of the bronchial tubes and prevents an attack. Although considered safe and effective, the medication gives only short-term relief and produces gastrointestinal or respiratory discomfort in about one out of eight patients.

The newest cortisone sprays have fewer side effects than the old ones, and bronchodilators (drugs that open the bronchial tubes and allow air to pass through) have improved in recent years, although a few cases of cardiac arrest and respiratory failure have been linked to extreme overuse of a popular inhaler called metaproteronol sulfate (brand name: Alupent).

Several nondrug approaches have surfaced as well. Scientists at the National Asthma Center in Denver researched the theory that it's not rapid breathing that triggers attacks in people who exercise, but the inhalation of cold air. When asthmatics wore simple face masks that warmed the air before it reached their lungs, they experienced many fewer attacks.

These and similar findings inspired commercial production of the Bodybreather, a runners' device that costs about $50; it is strapped to the chest and allows the wearer to breathe warm air from a plastic snorkel-like mouthpiece. *American Health* magazine (January/February 1983) tested the product and reported that users' "throat and lungs were grateful for the warmer air; chafed chests and egos were not." You can write for a brochure to the Xinox Corp , 85 Watermill Lane, Great Neck, NY 11021.

Another recent finding is that, contrary to previous thinking, exercise such as walking, swimming, dancing, and deep breathing can be beneficial to asthmatics. Walking, dancing, and deep breathing should be done only in clean, nonpolluted air, and swimming should be in a sheltered location. The warmth and humidity found around indoor pools eliminates the bronchospasms many patients get when they swim in cold, dry air.

A safe rule for asthmatics is to start exercise slowly, taking intermittent rest periods. Don't exceed your tolerance level, whether it's gentle knee bends or four sets of tennis. Stop at the first sign of a wheeze.

Some asthmatics have had good results with biofeedback, a technique that teaches control of involuntary muscles. Patients learn to relax and open up the bronchial tubes so that air can pass through freely. Biofeedback training can be expensive and requires time and concentration, but is often effective. (Biofeedback is discussed in more detail in Chapter 6.)

Other current treatments rely on air filters, careful food-elimination diets, and vitamin supplements; a recent study reported in *Tropical and Geographical Magazine* concluded that daily doses of one gram of vitamin C reduced the frequency of asthma attacks by 25 percent.

Saving Your Skin

Although many people feel that all skin disorders must be treated with medication, this may not be the case. Barring such complications as facial swelling or infection, poison oak and poison ivy will heal by themselves in two weeks and don't require treatment, medical or otherwise.

Several years ago the late natural-food proponent Euell Gibbons suggested that persons fearing exposure to poison ivy or poison oak could protect themselves by chopping up the leaves of these plants, mixing them with other foods, and eating them. He may have gotten the idea from those Native Americans who tried to desensitize their babies by giving them poison oak leaves to chew. The practice can cause complications, however, and is not recommended.

Desensitizing shots can be troublesome as well, and should not be used except by such persons as forestry workers or firefighters, whose livelihood depends on their being able to withstand exposure. A possible prevention method, aside from studying the plant's appearance to better avoid it, is to build up the body's tolerance with gradually increasing doses of poison oak or ivy antigen taken orally or injected intradermally. These must be started three to five months before exposure and will usually provide protection for six months to a year. See a dermatologist for this treatment, as most over-the-counter oral preparations are too weak to be effective.

New findings reject the old rule that you should wash the skin with strong soap and water immediately after exposure, because soap can spread the toxic oil called urushiol. A better treatment is to let a full force of cold water flow over the spot or area and then blot it dry with a clean towel, being careful not to let the used parts of the towel touch the rest of the body. This must be done as soon as possible—within an hour after contact. Once the skin has been washed, the rash is not contagious.

Dr. Vera Byers, wife of the male author of this book and also an immunologist, ran into a curious situation. "We were seeing a number of servicemen just back from Japan," she says, "and they all had poison oak in the same places—on their forearms and buttocks. We finally discovered it came from the lacquer the Japanese use on bar counters and toilet seats. The lacquer is made from the lac plant, which is akin to poison oak and ivy but not strong enough to sensitize the Japanese. The servicemen were already sensitized because of all the poison oak in America. When they leaned on the counters or sat on the toilet seats, their skin reacted to traces of urushiol in the lacquer."

Natalie Golos and Frances Golbitz, authors of *Coping with Your Allergies,* warn that persons sensitive to poison oak or ivy should probably avoid cashews, pistachios, and mangoes, members of the same biological family. The sticky sap on the skins of the plants contains the same urushiol. Yet many people who get poison oak or ivy can eat those foods with no problem. As stated earlier, biological food families are not infallible and may not require strict adherence.

Scientists have been able to turn off urushiol reactions within minutes in laboratory rabbits by using a special kind of antibody injection. They hope to have it perfected for humans by 1988. In the meantime, the medical treatment for poison oak and ivy remains Calamine lotion (to relieve itching), cortisone medications, and antihistamines—or just to leave it to time and nature.

A new treatment for eczema has garnered attention lately; Dr. David Horrobin of Nova Scotia claims to have found the first oral agent that is effective against the skin ailment suffered by 12 million Americans. The medication is evening primrose oil, an extract from the yellow flower that grows along the east coast of the United States and in Canada, and is sold in health-food stores as a nutrition booster.

The active ingredients are two essential fatty acids (acids that can't be formed in the body and must be provided by the diet) called linoleic and gamma-linoleic acid. In the body these convert into a substance called Prostaglandin E₁ (PGE₁), which plays a significant role in enhancing the immune system. Dr. Horrobin found primrose oil to be "effective against eczema in 90 percent of cases studied," but it is not known how many cases he studied. Dr. Michael Kaliner of the National Institute of Allergy and Infectious Diseases dismisses the claim as "unlikely." Time and further research will tell.

A better treatment, perhaps, is the Scotland Yard approach: find the culprit. If you have eczema, try these steps:

1. Play detective. A pretty 16-year-old had hand eczema that flared up whenever she had a date. Her parents told her it was nerves, but she suspected otherwise. On the advice of her doctor, she wrote down all the things she did on the days she was going out that weren't in her usual routine. The research paid off with the discovery that she curled her hair with setting lotion before a date, and her hands were reacting to a chemical in the lotion. When she substituted water, the rash cleared up.

2. Eliminate suspected foods or medication from your diet and avoid as many contactants as you can. Bring these substances back into your life one by one, watching to see which, if any, cause or aggravate the outbreak.

3. If you have hand eczema, protect yourself by putting on rubber gloves with cotton liners, and wear loose, preferably cotton clothing against other patches on the body. Heat can irritate eczema, so take lukewarm, not hot, baths or showers and skip strenuous exercise that causes you to perspire. Don't use soap, greasy cream, or over-the-counter salves.

4. If you fail to find a cause and the irritation persists, see a doctor for testing and possible short-term medication such as a mild (.1 percent concentration) steroid ointment. The same detection measures apply to hives.

For Insect Stings and Bites

The venom of individual insects has recently become available for diagnosis and desensitizing treatments, and is definitely advised if you're susceptible.

Some people find that taking 200 mg of vitamin B₁ (thiamine) a day gives the skin a slight odor that repels fleas, mosquitoes, and other insects. Large doses (three to ten grams) of vitamin C several days before exposure may also provide protection against a reaction.

If you're sensitive to insect bites or stings you should carry an emergency sting kit equipped with adrenalin. A new prescription product called the EpiPen Auto-Injector is easy to use. When you release the safety cap and press the device to your thigh (not your buttock), a dose of adrenalin is automatically injected. The kit also contains chewable antihistamine tablets, a tourniquet, and alcohol swabs. Check carefully with your doctor before considering the use of adrenalin, as it can be dangerous for patients with heart disease or hypertension.

For Cold and Heat Sensitivity

If you're a cold-sensitive Type 1, you can help yourself by observing a few commonsense rules. Sleep in a room heated to between 65 and 70 degrees, with the windows closed. Try to stay indoors on cool days; if you must go out, breathe through your nose so that the air can be warmed before it reaches your lungs. A cotton-gauze mask can help take the chill off the air you inhale. Avoid night swimming, picnics, barbecues, and other outdoor activities if you live in a cool climate, and don't drive in open convertibles. A strong wind can blow allergens such as dust and mold spores into your eyes, nose, and mouth, or the chill can push you over your tolerance threshold. Heat sensitivity is generally less prevalent and less acute, but Type 1 persons who have this symptom should also use common sense, dress in layers that can be shed, and avoid sunbathing and other activities that cause excess perspiring.

Some physicians have tried to desensitize patients to heat and cold by having them immerse their arms and legs in water of gradually increasing or decreasing temperature. Others suggest taking showers twice a day—one minute of hot water alternated with one minute of cold water for ten minutes—to accustom the body to temperature changes.

There have been no documented reports of success with these

techniques, and they could be dangerous, sending a sensitive person into anaphylactic shock. This causes the blood pressure to plummet, and suffocation and death may follow if the person is not treated promptly. The usual emergency procedure is a shot of adrenalin, which constricts blood vessels and raises blood pressure.

There is no medical treatment for heat and cold allergies except to get rid of such obvious allergens as pets, plants, and dust catchers, to reduce the total load of stresses on your body, and to raise your tolerance level.

Urine Autoinjection

This therapy was first introduced in 1947 and is enjoying a revival along with the current trend to "natural" remedies. It involves collecting and sterilizing the patient's urine and injecting it into the patient at intervals and in increasing strength. This type of treatment has a valid immunological basis in that many antigens are secreted in the urine; reintroducing them into the body can build up the population of T cells. But antigens from the kidneys are being reinjected at the same time, and can cause the immune system to start fighting off its own tissue. Because this can be extremely damaging to the kidneys, urine injection is a technique to avoid.

Pills, Drops, and Sprays: Not to Be Taken Casually

Medication is not the preferred treatment for Type 1 allergies, but it can slow reactions and provide relief. A wide variety of antihistamines is now available for specific allergic symptoms, and they are reasonably safe, effective drugs, in spite of a vast range of side effects. There are products to stop runny noses, to counteract motion sickness, to reduce the itching of hives, and to relieve stomach distress. Most of them put you to sleep, but some keep you awake. Most reduce your appetite, but some make you hungry. Most serve as depressants, but others stimulate. There are no general rules and no validity to advertising claims that some antihistamines make you less drowsy than others. A brand such as Actifed may slow down one person and excite another. It depends on many factors, starting with your genes.

These drugs are mainly beneficial to Type 1 persons with nose, eye, ear, throat, and skin problems, but they can also reduce symptoms caused by foods and chemicals. They generally help relieve hay fever but not asthma, hives but not contact eczema, and both seasonal and nonseasonal rhinitis.

A new kind of antihistamine, discovered in the early 1970s, blocks the action of histamine—the body substance that causes allergic reactions—in the stomach, and has the capacity to reduce secretion of gastric acids. Cimetidine (brand name: Tagamet), the first drug of this type to be sold in the United States, has become the best-selling medication in the country. Ulcer patients claim it has revolutionized their lives, and Type 1 persons occasionally take it for gastrointestinal symptoms.

Clinical ecologists prefer not to use any antihistamines, believing that drugs should be used only in life-threatening situations or so infrequently that the user doesn't develop a dependence on them. Thus the seasonal hay fever sufferer who can relieve simple pollen allergies with antihistamines once or twice a year should do so; there's no reason for medical treatment or drastic changes of lifestyle. However, if you feel you need chronic chemotherapy—that's the use of any drug, from aspirin on—consider trying diet control, environmental cleanup, and immunotherapy first.

Publicity and advertising campaigns often tout one antihistamine as "having fewer side effects" or as being "twice as effective" as other brands. Such claims are generally misleading and hard to prove.

In the fall of 1982 a large eastern drug company sent doctors across the nation a board game called "Journey Through Allergy Land," which promoted their brand of antihistamine. The game is clever and children may enjoy playing it, but the philosophy behind it is destructive; its depiction of the "High Pollen Count" as a wicked monster and the wind as a vicious creature who "turns loose large clouds of evil pollen to float through your head" is ill conceived. Reputable allergists don't say that pollens are bad in and of themselves—in fact, they're very beneficial and necessary—but only that if you're allergic to them you should not be around them. Trying to sell a drug or treat an illness by instilling fear and hatred is harmful and irresponsible.

The side effects of antihistamines include dryness of the mouth, nose, and throat; gastric distress; chills; confusion; nervousness; irritability; dizziness; euphoria; temporary impotence; increase in blood pressure; chest tightness; headache; constipation; blurred vision; palpitations; urinary problems; and sensitivity to light. Sometimes the pills bring on the very symptoms they're taken to cure: a stuffy nose, wheezing, a skin rash. Or they do exactly what they shouldn't do: thicken mucus and clog the nasal passages.

The point is that antihistamines are neither "non-habit-forming" nor "safe for everyone." A bank executive who took over-the-counter antihistamines whenever his backyard acacia bloomed had concurrent problems with insomnia. When he stopped taking the pills, he was able to sleep again, but he made no connection until some months later when he tried a new appetite suppressant and found that it kept him awake and jumpy all night. He discovered that both the appetite suppressant and the antihistamine contained phenylpropanolamine (PPA), a common decongestant that can raise blood pressure and, for some people, act as a central nervous system stimulant. When he discontinued the pills, he had no more problems.

Another example is a woman with respiratory symptoms who had been taking antihistamines three times a day for twelve years. She also had terrible body eczema that her internist was treating with prednisone, a powerful steroid. It was obvious from her personal history that constant exposure to dog dander was causing her congested nose and sore throat, and that the antihistamines she took to relieve these symptoms gave her a skin rash. A clinical ecologist, appalled at the idea of using one drug to treat the side effects of another, took her off all medication and convinced her to give away her beloved dachshund. Several months later the woman's health returned.

Many people who buy antihistamines, either over-the-counter or prescription, take too many or too strong a dosage. The bottle may say you can take up to four pills a day, and while that amount won't kill you it might turn you into a walking zombie. If you must take antihistamines, try half a pill the first time and see if it helps. Some people find that if they take antihistamines only when absolutely necessary, their bodies are freshly responsive to the medication, and the half dose is enough.

Continuous use of nasal sprays or drops can be an equally bad habit. They may be fine for occasional relief, but so many people overuse these drugs that doctors have given a name to this dependence: "rhinitis medicamentosa," or rebound phenomenon.

Here's what happens. You use the spray or drops, which shrink the swollen nose lining and clear the passages. Suddenly you can breathe again. Soon afterward, however, the body counteracts the drug effects by causing the nose to swell even more than before. You reach for your medicine and the cycle starts. The more you use the spray or drops, the more you swell, and soon the blockage becomes chronic. Bacteria and viruses get trapped in the thick, dry mucus and you become readily prone to infection.

Decongestants also damage the cilia—tiny, delicate hairs that filter dust, pollen, and other allergens out of the air you breathe. This negates an important defense mechanism and makes the allergic person more vulnerable to inhalants.

Most decongestants, especially nonprescription, contain a drug called phenylephrine that is very similar to the phenylpropanolamine in antihistamines. Both chemical components reduce congestion by contracting the small blood vessels in the nose, and act as stimulants that can cause nervousness, insomnia, and elevated blood pressure. These drugs put added stress on the body— exactly what the allergic person doesn't need.

The newest form of decongestant is made from steroids, synthetic hormones that are very effective in critical cases when used on a short-term basis closely supervised by a doctor. In noncritical patients, they'll reduce nasal swelling along with all other inflammation in the body, depriving you of an important defense against infection. Thus you not only become more susceptible to bacteria and viruses, but your body has no way of keeping the infection localized, so it spreads to other parts of the anatomy. Prolonged use of steroids can cause brittle bones, hair growth on face and body, cataracts, increased appetite, fluid retention, and a characteristic "moon face" or puffy look. Don't take steroids casually.

One possible alternative is deceptively simple and, for some people, surprisingly effective. Dr. Ben Robinson, a San Francisco psychiatrist, was searching for a nondrug way to help his wife, Gloria, who endured daily sneezing, coughing, and general allergic discomfort. A colleague suggested saline nose drops, a solution of salt and water in exactly the same proportion as normal body fluids.

Dr. Robinson bought some "sodium chloride irrigation solution" at the medical laboratory and gave it to Gloria to try. She found that by squirting a half-dropperful of the solution into each nostril morning and night she could loosen the clogged mucus, which then flowed into her mouth and had to be expectorated. The drops seemed to flood out the allergens stored in her nasal passages and clear her pathways for breathing. She felt great relief, and still treats herself twice a day.

"The advantage of saline drops," says Dr. Robinson, "is that there are no side effects. You're not taking a drug or introducing a substance that's foreign to the body. All you're doing is enhancing the drainage from the sinuses by increasing the flow of normal body fluid. It's best to take the drops lying down, or with your head way back over the side of your bed. You may want to heat the solution to body temperature. And there's no reason to go to a medical lab. You can make the drops at home by adding one-fourth teaspoon of salt to an eight-ounce glass of water."

Some doctors recommend a humidifier in the bedroom to keep the mucus thin and flowing, but you must clean the device daily so that mold doesn't grow in it. A number of physicians also advocate moderate amounts of vitamin A for building up cilia and stimulating the growth of healthy mucus-producing cells.

For Gastrointestinal Symptoms

Since food allergies are the prime cause of Type 1 stomach and intestinal disorders, the basic treatment is to eliminate the offending foods, as we will discuss in Chapter 4.

Traditional allergists may recommend taking antihistamines or cromolyn sodium, the drug used to prevent asthma attacks, before a possibly allergenic meal. In cases of acute cramping due to food allergy, doctors may administer a small subcutaneous (under the skin) injection of adrenalin.

For Cerebral Symptoms

Mental states such as gloominess, irritability, or giddiness that are related to Type 1 allergies almost always clear up when the physical symptoms are alleviated or when certain drugs, such as antihistamines, are discontinued.

Generally speaking, Type 1 patients have every reason for optimism. Diagnostic tools have been sharpened to provide easy identification of allergens, drug-free treatment techniques are improving daily, and environmental control is being enhanced by a constant stream of new products. Even more encouraging is the fact that Type 1 symptoms tend to diminish with the passing of time.

Type 2 allergies follow a very different pattern and offer challenges that human beings have never had to cope with before.

Chapter 3

PORTRAIT OF A TYPE 2

In 1977 Debra Lynn Dadd was a 22-year-old classical pianist who had just moved to a new apartment in San Francisco. It had wall-to-wall synthetic carpets, polyester drapes, and a splendid view of the Golden Gate Bridge. She noticed that the setting sun warmed up the drapes and made them smell "horrid." The kitchen had particle-board cabinets (formaldehyde resin), formica counters, and a soft linoleum floor. Sleeping quarters boasted a fireproofed foam mattress with Dacron pillow and polyester sheets. Fumes from the recently refinished piano filled the air.

Debbie's normal wake-up time was about seven A.M., but in the new surroundings she'd wake up at least half an hour later, very groggy, and then fall back to sleep. When she finally dragged herself out of bed, she'd take a shower, giving herself a good dose of chlorine vapors, and eat cereal and milk for breakfast while reading the morning paper, saturated with chemicals from the fresh newsprint.

By this time she was ready to go back to bed again. But she would force herself to dress in her mainly synthetic clothes, apply scented cosmetics and deodorant, and finally, at about eleven A.M., she would sit down to practice piano. After half an hour, she would need to go outside for a walk to clear her head.

She became engaged and started spending time at her fiancé's home. It was her first exposure to gas heating. To her surprise, whenever she went to see him she found herself quarreling with everything he said, crying uncontrollably, and often becoming hysterical. When she saw him anywhere else, they were fine. The strain of her unpredictable moods eventually became intolerable, and they agreed to call off the wedding.

Eating became obsessive, and she gained weight. Along with insomnia and constant fatigue, she experienced a lack of motivation and strong self-doubts. Much of the time she felt confused and spacey. Her father suggested that she see a clinical ecologist; tests for chemicals proved positive, but the antigens the doctor provided contained phenol and glycerin preservatives, and made her feel worse. No one suggested environmental changes, so the treatment failed.

A year later she went to see a new clinical ecologist who recognized the importance of cleaning up her surroundings. She soon began to see direct connections with her symptoms. If she stood near someone wearing perfume, for instance, her mind would "short-circuit," leaving her unable to concentrate or think. She also related a sharp rise in her pulse rate during her morning shower to the chlorine in the water—this after five days of a doctor-approved fast that made all her symptoms more acute.

The new approach called for changing her clothing and bedding to natural fibers, giving away scented cosmetics and cleaning products, and avoiding all reading material with fresh newsprint. Little by little she regained her health and her energy. Some time later she went into a home with gas heat and began to cry for no reason. It quickly became obvious why her temper tantrums had occurred only in her ex-fiancé's home.

Today Debbie considers herself "cured." She takes no medication and lives in an apartment with hardwood floors and cotton curtains, close to the ocean. Her work as the author's medical technician and researcher is challenging and stimulating, and, as long as she controls the environments where she spends most of her time, her Type 2 allergies cause no problems.

"I don't feel I'm being deprived," she says. "In fact, I think I'm living better. But I worry about the great numbers of people with chemical allergies who are still walking around undiagnosed. That's why it's important to know what symptoms to look for."

TYPE 2 SYMPTOMS

Mood and Behavior Changes

The most striking symptoms of Type 2 allergies are the cerebral and behavioral reactions. Depression, paranoia, extreme fatigue, hyperactivity, delusions, hallucinations, panic, amnesia, blackouts, and manic, phobic, and violent responses may all be linked to everyday substances that surround us. Somewhat milder symptoms include dizziness, confusion, irritability, lack of motivation, memory loss, unusual sensitivity to sounds and odors, a feeling of spaciness, slurred speech, difficulty in concentration, and minor personality changes.

It must be emphasized here that *not all cerebral symptoms are caused by allergies*. The traditional Freudian approach holds that mental illness is a result of the patient's genetic inheritance, childhood experiences, sexual development, and the stresses of living. Hereditary tendencies plus emotional strains can undoubtedly elicit symptoms ranging from mild depression to catatonic (comatose) schizophrenia.

But chemicals can affect the brain, too, and in many more ways than the average person realizes. Clinical ecologists estimate that at least seven out of ten people who have mental problems are allergic to foods, inhalants, or chemicals—or to all three—and that these allergies directly cause or intensify brain malfunctions. They're convinced that allergic reactions are one of the major causes of violence in America, having witnessed and treated thousands of cases of Type 2 "cerebral allergy"—patients previously diagnosed as neurotic or insane who did not respond to conventional therapies but who became miraculously "sane" in a matter of days. And the answer was often as simple as eliminating a food, a chemical, or a substance from the environment.

A recent case involved a 45-year-old FBI agent whose job took him all over the country. His health was perfect until he developed infectious hepatitis, and several months after his recovery he began to notice that he was afraid to fly in commercial airplanes. The moment the aircraft doors closed, he would feel strong forebodings, as if death were inevitable. He tried every sort of mental and psychological ploy to reduce his newly acquired fear, even going to see a psychiatrist, who diagnosed "phobic behavior" and warned about business stresses. The doctor prescribed tranquilizers and "several martinis" during the flight.

Fortunately, the man felt that his irrational fear must have other origins, and acted on a friend's suggestion that he try clinical ecology. Tests revealed sensitivity to formaldehyde and phenol, chemicals found in high concentrations in the closed environment of pressurized aircraft. The hepatitis had lowered his resistance and made him newly vulnerable to his latent chemical allergies.

Armed with this information, he began to clean up his surroundings and reduce his *total load*—the number of specific allergens and other chemicals in the environment that combine to weaken the immune system. (Chemicals are toxins as well as sensitizers.) He removed almost all synthetic materials from his bedroom and office, eliminated processed foods from his diet, and allowed his immune system to regain normal function, thereby raising his tolerance threshold. Three months later he was able to fly in airplanes with a minimum of fear and discomfort.

Another example is that of a 20-year-old guitarist classified as a paranoid schizophrenic. She sought treatment at the urging of her brother, who couldn't understand why she was perfectly sane much of the time but became "crazy" around their cigar-smoking neighbor.

The patient was taught to scrutinize her habits and her environment, recording everything she did and everyone she saw preceding a schizophrenic episode. Finally, the offending agents were narrowed down to diesel fumes, tobacco smoke, and perfumes. When she is away from these allergens, her "craziness" disappears.

A common cerebral symptom that is often difficult to explain is lethargy—lack of energy or ambition. As Debbie Dadd recalls, "It took a great deal of sleuthing to track this one down, but it's all true. A 31-year-old man came in with a long list of complaints, one of them being that he just couldn't get out of bed in the morning. We had him change his pillow, linens, even the bed itself, move out all plastic furniture, and sleep in a room with hardwood floors and the window open. Nothing. No improvement.

"But he noticed a very strange thing. If he got to sleep early and awoke naturally before seven A.M., he could bounce out of bed full of energy. If he awoke after seven he was groggy. Well, it turned out that the freeway was five blocks from his house and the fumes from the commuter traffic caused a reaction. The solution was to sleep with the window open all night but to close it before the traffic started at seven.

"I've gotten to know this man well and I've seen him yawn and get tired if even one car drives by. Maybe his tale will help some of those people who can't understand why they feel sleepy at the wheel. If they were to travel when the streets are relatively empty, avoid congested highways, and keep their windows closed in heavy traffic, they'd probably find that their sleepiness would disappear."

Children often have the opposite symptom—hyperactivity. The American Medical Association maintains that there's no proven connection between hyperactivity and allergy, particularly to foods, but any observant parent of a hyperactive child will tell you differently.

A television crew recently went to an environmentally oriented pediatrician's office and filmed a dramatic sequence. Two-year-old Ricky had regular temper tantrums. Everyone said he was spoiled, but his mother refused to accept that diagnosis. Previous tests had indicated a sensitivity to food coloring. Ricky chewed a piece of pink bubble gum and began to get irritable in twenty minutes. Within an hour, he was on the floor screaming and kicking. It took two people to hold open his mouth while the doctor squirted a neutralizing dose of red dye antigen under his tongue. His tantrum subsided within minutes.

Parents often have problems with children who become hyperactive in cars; they feel sick, nauseated, tense, cranky, and fatigued and constantly whine, complain, and cry. These might well be allergic reactions to exhaust fumes blowing into the back seat or to the plastic interior of the car.

Dr. Theron Randolph, the "father" of clinical ecology; Dr. Marshall Mandell; Dr. Joseph McGovern, Jr.; and many other physicians have documented case after case of cerebral allergy. Their writings are available; several are listed in the References section. Suffice it to say that mood and behavior changes are all Type 2 symptoms, and very different from Type 1 symptoms. A Type 1 person may feel depressed because pollens make his eyes itch and his nose run; his gloom accompanies his allergy. A Type 2 person's depression, in contrast, is an allergic symptom itself, a direct brain response to any or to many of a wide variety of substances.

Mainly Migraines

Scientists are beginning to recognize that a vast number of neurological (as well as psychological) ailments are not caused by emotional states, but are actual allergies that affect the brain.

The sinus headache previously mentioned was a Type 1 symptom. The tension or muscle spasm headache is a similar dull pressure in the front or back of the head, slightly higher than the sinus headache, and on both sides rather than only on one. It rarely throbs, is not associated with nasal congestion, and is very common among Type 2 persons.

Not quite so common, fortunately, are the dreaded migraines. Yet these afflict 38 million Americans, according to June Biermann and Barbara Toohey, authors of *The Woman's Holistic Headache Relief Book*. The throbbing pain is caused by an enlargement of blood vessels that press against delicate nerves, and can last up to forty-eight hours. Migraines, which affect more women than men, are associated with stress, weather changes, amounts of sleep, loud noises, bright lights, high altitudes, and occasionally Type 1 inhalants such as dust and pollens.

Most migraines, however, are related to Type 2 sensitivities to foods, odors, natural gas, chemical fumes, and hormonal changes. Pregnancy, menstruation, and menopause seem to be closely linked to migraine symptoms, and Dr. Lee Kudrow of the California Medical Clinic for Headache found an unusually high incidence of migraines in women using oral contraceptives or taking estrogens. Stopping birth-control pills reduced the frequency and intensity of migraines for 70 percent of the women he studied.

In another study, Dr. John Mansfield, a British clinical ecologist, found that wheat, oranges, eggs, tea, coffee, chocolate, milk, beef, corn, cane sugar, yeast, mushrooms, and peas—in declining order—were the most common migraine producers. Among patients who excluded these foods from their diet, 85 percent suffered no more headaches and the rest experienced a significant lessening of pain.

Tyramine—an organic compound that swells the blood vessels in the head—is known to specifically provoke migraines. Tyramine is found in most cheeses, chicken and beef livers, pickled herring, cured meats, caviar, chocolate, yogurt, broad beans, red wine, and imported beers.

Authors Biermann and Toohey tabulated the findings of several doctors and came up with a list of the top headache (both migraine and muscle spasm) producers, in order of importance: milk, chocolate, eggs, wheat, peanuts, citrus fruit (including tomatoes), and pork. Obviously, if you are a headache sufferer you do not have to avoid all these foods, but at least you should have a good idea what to suspect, and when you start the Food Sensitivity Diet in Chapter 4 you'll know which foods to test first.

As with all baffling allergic symptoms, one must play detective. Take the example of a 38-year-old engineer who suddenly started getting migraines and short-term memory loss for no apparent reason. He had been working for years in a drafty old warehouse where the windows wouldn't close properly. There was tension in the office and the hours were long, but he loved the work and was happy.

His wife, however, was not. She pressed him to take a job with a large company where he would have regular hours and more time to spend with his family. So he moved to a new position in a new office in a highrise building. His old wooden desk and drafty room with the cracked plaster were replaced by streamlined vinyl furniture, a controlled temperature and environment, and synthetic drapes and carpets.

The moment he walked into the building he was hit with a wall of chemicals. Within five minutes his head would begin to throb and he would forget such trivial things as where he had put his keys or his pen. A supervisor diagnosed "job burnout" and sent him to a company psychiatrist, who prescribed tranquilizers and painkillers.

When his problems became worse, he found his way to our office, where tests showed allergies to formaldehyde and other chemicals that abound in new buildings. He got rid of his synthetic furnishings, installed an air filter, and made himself take ten-minute "air breaks"—walking in the fresh breeze—every hour. His headaches and other symptoms gradually subsided.

If you're considering medical care for this problem, you can speed the doctor's diagnosis by writing out a description of your headache symptoms:

1. Is it dull and constant or does it throb?
2. Is it better when you lie down or stand up?
3. Is it in the front part of your head or in the back? On one side or both sides?

4. Do you get any warning signs?
5. What other symptoms are associated with it? Dizziness? Nausea? Stomach cramps? Changes in vision? Stuffy nose? Confusion?
6. How often do you get one?
7. Does it last for minutes, hours, or days?
8. Does it come at the same time of day?
9. Does it come at special times of the month or year?
10. What medication helps?

Each answer provides a clue. Throbbing, for instance, is generally associated with migraines but can also be a sign of hypertension. If you have a dull, constant headache for long periods of time, a brain tumor must be considered, although it's very unlikely. A headache that's worse when you're lying down also indicates the remote possibility of a brain tumor.

The location supplies more pieces of the puzzle. Migraines are freqently one-sided, near the temple, behind the eye, or over the ear. Muscle-tension headaches are usually on top or toward the back of the head. You can have both kinds of headaches at once or intermittently.

The warning signs of a migraine are mainly visual changes: flashing lights, wavy lines on walls, blurring, and blind spots. Chills, disorientation, loss of appetite, vomiting, diarrhea, and shoulder and back pains may also accompany migraines. Dizziness would more likely be associated with a middle-ear problem, viral infection, or hypertension.

Frequency of occurrence tells the doctor what kind of treatment is needed. If you get a classic migraine every six months and can relieve it with medication, you don't need to restrict your diet, change your environment, or spend more money on medical bills. You can get along fine with two pills a year. If you suffer migraines three or four days a month, however, you need immediate treatment.

A headache that recurs at a specific hour every morning is a good clue. Look at your environment. Are there machines or appliances that are turned on at certain times of day? Do you take a coffee break at ten A.M. or eat peanuts at three in the afternoon?

Do you reach for the phone at nine? See a particular person at four? The time of month or year your headaches appear could indicate a relation to menstruation, to the mold or pollen season, or to certain foods such as cranberries that are eaten mainly on holidays.

It is vital to your health to recognize and understand muscle-tension headaches, migraines, and all characteristic Type 2 reactions. Many physicians, faced with an array of seemingly unrelated symptoms and unaware of the role of chemicals in causing disease, misdiagnose these ailments as "psychosomatic," "nerves," or hysteria. In a sincere attempt to help the patient, they recommend psychotherapy or prescribe strong drugs, failing to realize that there may be a simple, removable cause.

The following symptoms are those most often associated with Type 2 allergies: changes of mood and behavior, headaches, palpitations, blurred vision, feeling spacey, numbness, fatigue, generalized itching, burning or flushing of the skin, muscle and joint aches, gastrointestinal upsets, food and alcohol addiction, and specific cravings for food, alcohol, and tobacco. (Obesity, alcoholism, and addiction are discussed in the next chapter.)

Many health problems such as arthritis, colitis, gall bladder disorders, epilepsy, depression, schizophrenia, multiple sclerosis, systemic lupus erythematosus, and some forms of cancer are now known to be clearly related to Type 2 allergies. Undoubtedly, your next question is: What causes all these symptoms? And the answer is right before your eyes in the form of synthetic chemicals, air pollution, certain foods, and some other substances you've probably never thought about.

TYPE 2 ALLERGENS

The human organism, in common with all of life, is chemically constituted and lives in an environment that is likewise 100 percent chemical. Barring all synthetic materials, our "natural" environment would still be wholly chemical.

It is unfair and simplistic to equate the word "chemical" with "toxic" in all instances. Synthetic compounds, fibers, and fabrics are mainly responsible for our high standard of living. In the small

republic of Togo on the west coast of Africa, where the inhabitants
have no sanitation facilities, no sewage or garbage disposal systems, no water-purification techniques, no modern medicines, and
almost no chemical technology of any sort, the average life span is
thirty-eight years.

It may help to keep perspective if we note that the role of
environmental pollutants as an unseen form of illness is exactly the
same as the role of germs in illness that Louis Pasteur pointed out
over a century ago. Germs then were as invisible as chemicals are
today, and caused an equal amount of controversy. In the next
century, there will surely be something else.

Nevertheless, the problem exists. Over many centuries, our
bodies have miraculously evolved to tolerate or require most of the
naturally occurring substances that surround us. Yet there are
many synthetic substances in our environment to which our bodies
have not had sufficient time to adapt. At the present moment
we're being exposed to concentrations of these chemicals that are
ten to a hundred times higher than those with which our ancestors
lived, and which tax our adaptive mechanisms to their maximum.

Our bodies' struggle to deal with all these agents often leads
to breakdowns in our immune system. Such malfunctions show up
as mild, acute, or chronic Type 2 allergic reactions.

Chemical sensitivity is the resultant illness, and it can be
defined as an intolerance to specific chemicals in the everday environment. This uniquely Type 2 ailment has many names: environmental illness, chemical allergy, chemical susceptibility, cerebral
allergy, and ecologic or bioecologic illness. Some even call it
"hives on the brain."

The questionnaire in Chapter 1 referred to such environments
as a traffic jam or an energy-sealed office building that are particularly heavy with chemical fumes and likely to provoke Type 2
symptoms. But even our everyday environment abounds in synthetic chemicals.

In a typical household on an average morning, typical people
wake up on synthetic foam-rubber mattresses snuggled between
cotton-polyester sheets and acrylic blankets, clothed in nylon
sleepwear, their heads resting on Dacron pillows.

When they arise, their feet touch the polypropylene carpet as
they walk to open the rayon drapes. They move to a chair padded
with polyurethane and covered with polyvinyl, put on their drip-

dry robes and acrylic slippers and patter to the bathroom. There they brush their teeth with plastic toothbrushes, using artificially colored and flavored toothpaste. Hot water fills the air with chlorine fumes mingled with the perfumed scents of the soap, shampoo, and plastic shower curtain. She applies some chemical dyes to her face, he "purifies" his breath with aerosol spray.

They dress in polyester, mothproofed wool, and no-iron cotton and then sit down to breakfast. The eggs, sizzling in a Teflon pan, are full of hormones; the butter has been dyed yellow; the bacon is preserved in nitrites; the grapefruit was grown with synthetic pesticides and fertilizers; the English muffins have been processed with flavorings, extenders, and emulsifiers; and they've all been packaged in polyethylene and stored in refrigerators insulated with polyurethane and cooled by chlorofluorocarbons. What a mouthful—literally!

They then drive to work in a car loaded with synthetic rubber, plastic, and polyurethane, powered by gasoline. And so it goes. Life without synthetics would be unimaginable.

Fortunately, most of these compounds do not bother most people, but the number of chemically sensitive patients is growing at an alarming rate. This is mainly due to the process of *outgassing*—that is, the giving off of gases. Seemingly inert materials such as plastic or synthetic fibers all have volatile components that evaporate slowly and constantly, emitting undetectable fumes into the air.

Over twenty-five years of clinical experience have identified the compounds that do the most damage to the immune system and cause the greatest number of Type 2 reactions. "Immunotoxic" chemicals fall into four main categories:

1. *Petrochemicals*. These are compounds created from prehistoric plant and animal life. Millions of years of underground processing by extreme heat and pressure have produced a product that in solid form is coal and asphalt, in liquid form is petroleum or crude oil, and in gaseous form is natural gas. Many everyday products come from these sources: perfume, food dyes and additives, synthetic fibers, plastic, alcohol, paints, inks, adhesives, cleaning solvents, and countless other items. Even the candles on your dining room table are made from paraffin derived from petroleum, and are colored with petroleum dyes.

Formaldehyde, a petrochemical derivative, is said to be the

most common chemical in the average household. It is used as an antiperspirant, antiseptic, disinfectant, preservant, and explosive, and it helps make fabrics flameproof, mothproof, waterproof, wrinkleproof, and shrinkproof. When smog burns your eyes, blame formaldehyde. Petrochemicals are everywhere.

2. *Halogens*. The most common form of halogens is chlorine. It does not occur freely in nature but is part of many compounds, such as the familiar sodium chloride, or salt. Halogens also appear in paper pulp, insect killers, herbicides, anesthetics, drugs, and processed foods.

3. *Sulfur*. Relatively nontoxic in its natural state, sulfur can cause problems when it reaches us in the form of air pollution, medication, metal polish, photographic supplies, dandruff shampoo, food preservatives, and sulfur dioxide, found in almost all wine.

4. *Ammonia*. This is usually synthesized from petrochemical derivatives and is found in such products as disinfectants, additives in bakery goods, glues, fertilizers, fabric dyes, rubber, soap, rayon, refrigerants, and urea formaldehyde foam, a common home-insulating material.

These four categories are like the biological food families in that an allergy to the chemical in any one product may indicate a sensitivity to all associated products. If you're bothered by the chlorine in swimming pools, for instance, you should think twice before adding bleach to your laundry.

The greatest menace to Type 2 persons are the fumes from elements found indoors, where the typical American spends 90 percent of each day. According to a study done by the National Aeronautics and Space Administration, even woods and metals give off gases to some degree. Here is NASA's list of the outgassing capacity of common materials, listed in decreasing order, starting with polyesters, which outgas the most:

Polyesters	Aluminum
Polyethylenes	Copper
Polyvinyls	Hardwood
Silicones	Iron
Epoxies	Steel
Polyurethanes	Ceramic
Fluorocarbons	Stone

Dr. Phyllis Saifer, a clinical ecologist in Berkeley, California, and her husband, biophysicist Mark Saifer, have prepared another list that gives the most common sources of the seven top NASA offenders:

Polyesters: fabrics for clothing, upholstery, drapery, and bedding; stuffing for pillows, quilts, furniture, and winter garments.

Polyethylenes: food and milk containers.

Polyvinyls: shower curtains, leatherette upholstery, artificial flowers, gas and water pipes, and electrical conduits.

Silicones: used as a sealant to keep water out of dishwashers, washing machines, refrigerators, and all other major appliances.

Epoxies: adhesives on plastic articles and on electronic equipment such as home computers, television sets, and microwave ovens.

Polyurethanes: pillows, mattresses, furniture stuffing, and building insulation.

Fluorocarbons: Teflon utensils and the freon gas that leaks from refrigerators and freezers.

The Saifers have added to the list of common indoor pollutants:

Building materials: brick, concrete, and granite can emit radioactive radon gas.

Car exhaust: from cars stored in garages.

Chlorine: in tap water, bath water, dishwashers, toilet bowls, and bleach.

Fireplaces: ink fumes from burning newspapers and other objects, preservatives used to treat wood, and synthetic logs.

Formaldehyde: plywood, paper products, fabric finishes, air deodorizers, and many other products.

Inks: in newsprint, books, and felt-tip markers.

Natural gas: stoves, furnaces, clothes dryers, and water heaters. (Dr. Frank E. Speizer of Harvard University Medical School studied 8,000 children and found that those who lived in homes with gas stoves suffered up to 15 percent more respiratory illnesses than those whose parents cooked with electricity.)

Pesticides: on pets and in foods, fumigants, and mothproofing.

Paint: stored in cans not tightly sealed.

Smoke: cigarettes, cooking.

Woods: used in home construction, furniture, and flooring. Soft woods such as fir, cedar, redwood, and pine have resins or terpenes (Christmas tree odor) that can outgas for years.

Many Type 2 symptoms, including headaches, make a dramatic first appearance after some type of insult to the body. It could be a short-term exposure to high concentrations of toxic materials from an industrial accident, or it could be long-term exposure to lesser concentrations from a poorly ventilated home or office. Other factors that can bring on Type 2 symptoms are psychological stress and severe viral attacks such as mononucleosis, influenza, or hepatitis.

Heat should be mentioned here, even though it is not strictly a Type 2 allergen. It can, however, change a substance into a more allergenic form. All synthetic products, such as clothing, furnishings, cosmetics, and cleaning solvents, may begin to outgas when exposed to heat. The summer sun beating down on tars and asphalt in roads and rooftops also increases outgassing.

A final allergen is *Candida albicans,* a common yeast that lives in the gut of every human being as a natural intestinal flora. It can cause a progressive condition called candidiasis, occasionally seen in Type 1 patients but more commonly associated with Type 2s.

Several years ago an Alabama internist, Dr. C. Orian Truss, made a startling discovery. A 40-year-old woman patient was suffering from depression, migraine headaches, and chronic yeast (monilia or *Candida albicans*) infection in the vagina. When he treated her experimentally with a neutralizing shot of Candida extract, her headache and depression cleared miraculously.

A second woman came to see him. Her psychiatrist had diagnosed her as a schizophrenic and recommended that she be institutionalized. The woman had a severe case of yeast vaginitis after taking antibiotics for a respiratory infection, and did not respond to the usual suppository treatment. So Dr. Truss gave her an oral antifungus agent called nystatin. To his surprise, not only did the vaginal infection clear up but so did the psychiatric symptoms. Her normal mental state lasted about two weeks, when her vaginitis recurred and, with it, the schizophrenia. Dr. Truss again treated her with nystatin, and again both her infection and her psychosis vanished.

After many more experiments, he reached this conclusion: Our bodies are engaged in a lifelong struggle with *Candida albicans*. As a foreign substance, its growth is controlled by the immune system. When some outside agent such as viral disease, stress, high chemical exposure, or a drug (cortisone, antibiotics, the birth-control pill) alters the immune system, we become hypersensitive to our own Candida and experience symptoms such as depression or mental disorders. It's as if a person allergic to pine has a pine tree growing right inside his nose.

As of this writing, there is no valid procedure to detect allergic candidiasis. Provocative testing may indicate a sensitivity to Candida, but does not necessarily mean that the patient has the acute condition. So the doctor must rely on the patient's symptoms and medical history. Certainly recurrent yeast infections such as monilial vaginitis should arouse suspicion. The only way to make a positive diagnosis of candidiasis is to treat the patient for it and see if symptoms diminish.

TESTING, TESTING

If you were never before aware of Type 2 allergies and their influence on health and behavior, you may never have suspected the reason for your physical or mental problems. Now that you are aware, you may want confirmation. An orthodox practitioner does not test for chemicals and may even diagnose you as "nonallergic" because you don't react to skin tests for dust, pollen, or cat hair. If you get a mild reaction to an inhalant, he may start you on shots that contain phenol and glycerin preservatives, which—if you're chemically sensitive—could make you worse.

Only a clinical ecologist tests for chemical allergies. He will take a detailed medical history, examine you physically, and, if the facts warrant, suggest provocative testing with tiny sublingual doses of antigens. This must be done in a clean-air office under close supervision. If your reactions are generally mild ones, you may want to first test yourself at home. It could be risky, so be sure to get your doctor's okay.

Home Testing: The Sniff Test

In the At-Home Sniff Test, your first step is to take six glass jars with tight lids. Place a swatch of polyester or any synthetic fabric in the first, a few mothballs in the second, and cotton balls in the remaining four jars. Have a friend or spouse pour your favorite cologne into jar four and some alcohol into jar five, leaving jar six untouched. Seal the lids tightly and let them sit for three days.

Before you start the actual test, have alkali salts at the ready— either two Alka-Seltzer Gold tablets, or make your own by adding two tablespoons of baking soda and one tablespoon of potassium bicarbonate (available at pharmacies) to a pint of water. Alkali salts help neutralize the body acids produced in an allergic reaction, but they're not advised for persons with heart or kidney problems or high blood pressure, or for anyone on a low-salt diet. Two tablespoons of milk of magnesia can be used instead.

The next step is to take all six jars into a room with cross ventilation or, better yet, outdoors. Do this early in the morning, before eating, and when you're free of symptoms. Have someone with you at all times during the test to observe any reactions and to record your pulse rate.

Put the jars in front of you, close your eyes, and mix them up—then take one. Keep your eyes shut so that you don't know which jar you're testing. Hold it at arm's length from your face, open it, and sniff *very* cautiously. If you get no reaction, slowly bring the jar closer and inhale again. Wait at least fifteen minutes, sitting quietly. Don't read or write, as this would introduce other possible allergens. Your companion can read a book or magazine that's not freshly printed if he sits at least eight feet away. Check your pulse at five-minute intervals. A jump of ten or more points means you may be responding.

If you do get a reaction such as a headache, nausea, dizziness, change of mood, or palpitations, immediately shut the jar, stop testing, and leave the area. Take the alkali salts or the milk of magnesia. One to three grams of vitamin C may help. If you can, take a walk in fresh air and breathe deeply.

Do no more than one jar a day, and when you finish the first five chemicals, try five more products such as hair shampoo, kitchen cleanser, a plastic bag, a ball-point pen, or your favorite cosmetic.

Lab Testing

1. *The T and B Blood Cell Count and Helper/Suppressor Ratios T Cell Subsets.* Don't let the name scare you. This new lab technique does not detect specific allergies but records the severity of a patient's response by counting and comparing the number of T and B cells. If the T cell count drops below normal, or there are too many of one type of cell and not enough of another, this means the immune system is struggling and showing signs of stress. In severe cases, the count may show that the immune system is barely functioning at all.

The value of this test is that it confirms (or doesn't confirm) the diagnosis of immune dysregulation and lets the doctor know how much strengthening, if any, the immune system needs. It can apply to Type 1 patients, but clinical ecologists generally use it for their most unresponsive-to-treatment or puzzling Type 2 patients.

2. *The Cytotoxic Test.* You may have seen newspapers ads touting the "diagnose-all" of the 1980s—the "miracle test" that determines all your food and chemical allergies from a single drawing of blood.

Cytotoxic literally means "having a bad effect upon cells," and the technique is to take a blood sample and count the number of white cells present on a microscope slide before and after the addition of a weak solution of antigen. If the antigen destroys white cells, the substance is said to be allergenic.

Like the RAST, the cytotoxic test is convenient for the patient and sometimes useful when provocative testing causes too much discomfort. The test has a solid biochemical rationale, but depends on subjective judgments of the technicians and widely differing lab

techniques. Continued retesting may produce some common conclusions, but in general the results are unreliable.

Office Testing

1. *The Provocative-Neutralization (P-N) Sublingual Test.* The
tester squirts drops of the antigen under your tongue, where they
are immediately absorbed into the appropriate cells. You count to
30 and then swallow. The double goal of this technique is to find
the substances to which you're allergic and to establish the specific
concentration of allergen that clears your symptoms and provides
relief.

As with P-N intradermal testing, the technician supplies a
sheet of paper on which you record how you feel before you start.
Results are based strictly on your reactions, so it's important that
you be relatively symptom-free. The doctor has already told the
technician what substances to try. If you think your expectations
could influence your response, ask for a blind test; that means
you'll either get a placebo or an antigen, and you won't know
which is which.

At the end of a ten-minute period, you're given a higher or
lower dilution, and so on until the exact dosage that stops your
symptoms is found. This must be done for each substance to which
you react. The procedure can take several days or more.

Under strictly controlled office conditions, neutralizing works
for 95 percent of Type 2 patients. The 5 percent who can't be
switched off are usually people whose systems are overloaded with
chemicals. If they breathe fresh air for two or three months, clean
up their environment, and greatly decrease their chemical exposure, they can almost always be retested and neutralized.

The initial workup in a clinical ecologist's office may take several days. But once a patient is tested, he doesn't need to be
treated for or even avoid all the substances to which he's allergic.
The more he can improve his diet and clear the environment of
toxins, the more he reduces his total load—and the higher his level
of tolerance. That means he can endure many more allergens without reacting.

Conventionalists often argue that responses to P-N testing are
subjective and psychological. Ecologists counter by showing that
the same responses can be reproduced time and time again in

blind studies—that it, experiments where the subject is unaware of which substances he's being tested for and sometimes even unaware that he's being monitored.

Traditional allergists find the idea of neutralization "appealing" but claim that studies have not been sufficiently documented. If they were to spend an hour in a clinical ecologist's testing room, they might feel differently.

Two incidents that occurred during routine office procedures were particularly convincing. One concerned a middle-aged woman who was given, in a blind test, an extract of glycerin. It took only four minutes for her to go into a complete catatonic trance. A less concentrated dose of the same extract relieved her symptoms and brought her out of her stupor twelve minutes later. The idea that a common ingredient in perfume can turn a person's psychosis on and off like a light bulb is understandably difficult for most people, including doctors, to accept.

The second incident was no less dramatic. A young man walked into the office and said he "felt okay." He had a mild headache, but he had lived with it so long that he'd begun to accept it as normal. His first test was a dose of ethanol, ordinary alcohol. Three minutes later, he almost jumped off his chair. "My God," he cried, "what did you give me? I feel great! I haven't felt this good in years!"

What happened was most unusual: the technician had hit exactly the right dose with the first try. It neutralized and cleared up the chronic headache the patient hadn't realized he had. Subsequent testing confirmed his sensitivity to ethanol. He learned to recognize the many everyday items that contain it, such as aftershave lotion, inks, and detergents. He cut his exposure to these materials to a minimum and was soon able to live without the dull pain that had plagued him for years. No further treatment was needed.

2. *The Muscle Test.* This method, favored by chiropractors, is called *applied kinesiology.* The practitioner first establishes muscle strength by measuring, for instance, how readily the patient lifts a fifty-pound weight. An allergen is introduced and the muscles are again measured. If there is less resistance, the assumption is that the weakening of muscle power indicates an allergic reaction. The test is hampered, at present, by a lack of accurate measuring tools.

Whatever means you use to discover your allergies, that's only the first step in the process. Now comes the real challenge: What can you do about them?

NEW TREATMENTS FOR TYPE 2 PERSONS

The most recent developments in treating Type 2 allergies can be divided into two categories: specific and nonspecific. Specific therapy, as its name implies, has a particular effect on a particular group of T cells. Nonspecific therapy attempts to build up the immune system as a whole.

Specific Therapies

Antigen Therapy. After testing, the doctor will send you home with one or several bottles of antigens containing extracts specific to your sensitivities. Be sure to wait forty-eight hours before using them, as your body is full of allergens from the testing; adding more too soon might push you over your tolerance level. The drops may alleviate your symptoms, but consider them only as Band-Aids: they cover the damage but can't repair it. The only thing that will allow a chemically injured immune system to heal is to remove the chemicals.

Antigens can speed the process, however, by building up groups of T cells and making you more resistant to various substances. Sublingual drops perform the same function as desensitizing shots. The main advantage, along with the fact that the drops work more efficiently and can be easily self-administered, is that, for many patients, drops can turn off an allergic reaction as well as prevent it.

The treatment is safe for most people because the antigens are not physiologically addictive the way some medicines are, and you don't need to keep increasing the dosage to gain benefits. Some hypersensitive patients react to the preservatives in the drops and require special extracts that are 100 percent pure and are extremely perishable if they are not frozen between applications.

Standard treatment is to squirt a measured amount under the tongue once or twice every day, although you can use the drops up to four times a day if you need them to relieve acute symptoms. As stated earlier, the dilution and dosage must be precise, the timing must be right, and you must treat yourself for the exact substance to which you're reacting. If you take antigen for the glycerin in perfume when you're responding to the chlorine in water, you won't be relieved.

Once you start daily antigen therapy, you should sense improvement within two to four weeks, and response should be at its peak in six to eight months. After about a year, depending on the individual, doctors suggest a weaning process—a gradual reduction in the frequency of doses as long as symptoms don't recur. Some patients maintain their tolerance on one or two dosages a week; others find that the combination of avoidance and antigen therapy builds up such a strong immune system that they can stop treatment altogether two years after they started.

Another benefit is that once you build up your immunity to several substances, your tolerance level rises and you can stand exposure to other allergens, including foods, that you couldn't tolerate before.

Antigen therapy to desensitize for foods is a long-term, touchy treatment; a wrong dose can provoke severe symptoms, so many doctors avoid it. They will, however, provide antigens (particularly wheat, corn, or milk) for hypersensitive persons to use in case of unexpected exposure.

Some patients ask: "Since I'm allergic to oranges and you can turn off my symptoms with a dose of orange antigen, why can't I turn them off myself with a few drops of real orange juice?" We explain that they could indeed switch off their symptoms if they had the proper concentration of juice and the exact amount at the ready, but it's impossible to prepare the precise dosage outside of a laboratory because of the variables of natural products and conditions.

Nystatin. The specific treatment for candidiasis, a disease caused by allergic sensitivity to normal body flora, is nystatin, a drug that selectively destroys *Candida albicans* with minimal effect on beneficial flora. It is taken orally, in powder or pill form, starting with a tiny amount that "tapers up" to the therapeutic dose. In the first week, the patient often notices an increase of symptoms. This is a good sign, indicating that the organisms are dying rapidly and secreting their toxins into the system in high concentration. This phase soon passes and the patient feels better. If he has no reaction or no relief of symptoms after three weeks, he's assumed not to have allergic candidiasis, and the therapy is discontinued. The patient will have no side effects from the drug, 99.9 percent of the time.

In the last few years clinical ecologists have been treating patients with nystatin for a variety of diseases, including schizophrenia, severe depression, arthritis, skin rashes, and gastrointestinal ailments. About 30 percent show significant benefit.

It's only very recently that allergic candidiasis has been known to cause emotional disorders. Although it may seem strange that the treatment of a body mold can cure such diverse illnesses as schizophrenia and arthritis, when they are considered in terms of their basic biochemical mechanisms they are revealed to be quite similar diseases. The only difference, in fact, is the target organ for the immune response.

Since yeast feeds on carbohydrates, clinical ecologists often augment nystatin treatment with a low-carbohydrate diet that excludes highly refined foods such as sugar, white flour, white rice, and carbonated and alcoholic beverages. They might also recommend a Mold and Yeast-Free Diet (see Chapter 4 for details) that eliminates vinegar, cheese, mushrooms, dried fruit, and all fermented brews. Of course, it's impossible to avoid eating molds; chances are your plain broiled hamburger comes from a cow fed on a mold-derived antibiotic such as penicillin. But even if you don't eliminate molds completely, at least you'll be ingesting them in lesser amounts.

Patients are generally advised to help the body maintain its normal intestinal flora with supplements of Acidophilus, Theradophilus, or Lactinex in liquid, pill, or granule form, and to take 50 milligrams of each B vitamin a day. These should come from a yeast-free source such as rice, and this fact must be so indicated on the container.

The good news about allergic candidiasis is that once you get rid of it, your immune system becomes fortified and can usually keep the growth down for a long period. If it does come back, a short course of nystatin will check it. Be sure to note that this treatment is (1) safe but still experimental and (2) not a panacea for all food and chemical allergies that lead to mental disorders.

LaPacho Tea. This is a very new and scientifically untested treatment for candidiasis, mentioned here because some chemically sensitive patients are trying it and claiming "amazing" results. The tea is brewed from the inner bark of the Brazilian LaPacho, a tree strangely resistant to molds, and is sipped daily, or in some cases used as a vaginal douche. There is no clinical evidence to support any claims for its healing properties.

Nonspecific Therapies

Transfer Factor. A well-tested and clinically proven new allergy therapy, transfer factor is a material extracted from the white blood cells of healthy donors. Unlike antigens, which provide immunity to specific substances, transfer factor and other nonspecific therapies build the whole immune system so that the body can tolerate all allergens.

When transfer factor is taken from the blood of one person and injected, the recipient acquires the donor's tolerances and immunities. The material has been ultra-screened and filtered in the laboratory so that it cannot pass along the donor's viruses, such as hepatitis.

But there are drawbacks. Transfer factor is expensive to process; each injection costs about $150 and must be given every two weeks for six weeks. If it seems to be working, the treatment continues for six months, when a weaning is attempted. Transfer factor is not like insulin, which requires lifetime dependency. A patient should not need these injections for more than two years, at the maximum.

The medication has limited availability because the raw materials required for its manufacture are scarce. Also, transfer factor's side effects could cause heart or muscle malfunction, inflict temporary or permanent brain damage, and aggravate vasculitis, a condition of enlarged blood vessels. While such side effects are very rare, they make doctors reluctant to use transfer factor except as a last resort for Type 2 patients with grave and incapacitating symptoms.

In the last thirteen years, we've given it to over 300 such patients. Four percent became worse and had to stop the treatment, 28 percent reported no change, and 68 percent showed definite improvement. Blood tests corroborated the results. Transfer factor has been almost miraculous for some patients who have tried everything else, and it's constantly being improved and perfected.

Interferon. Interferon is a drug that may or may not live up to its premature raves. A natural protein produced by white cells, interferon has been called the body's Paul Revere. When virus, disease, or allergens attack, interferon spreads the word to cells throughout the immune system to alert them to start producing antibodies.

Enthusiasts say this drug will cure everything from cancer to varicose veins, including herpes. Some maintain it increases the activity of T cells. Others believe that the interferon molecule contains components of transfer factor and therefore will prove to be even more effective than transfer factor in controlling allergies. All claims have yet to be proven.

The National Institute of Allergy and Infectious Diseases has been studying interferon since 1981, but reports that research is still in its infancy, and it may be years before this drug becomes available to the public. At least fifteen pharmaceutical firms have invested huge sums in interferon research on the assumption that natural body chemicals will be the drugs of tomorrow.

Thymosin. Thymosin, another natural body substance (extracted from the thymus gland of cows), belongs to a family of hormones that regulate the growth and maturation of the immune system. Although still under study, thymosin injections are being used in more than 150 hospitals and medical centers to enhance the body's natural defense network, particularly in cases of rheumatoid arthritis, multiple sclerosis, systemic lupus erythematosus, cancer, and a wide spectrum of allergies. Reports of success are as yet undocumented.

Propanolol. Propanolol (trade name: Inderal), a drug mainly used to treat heart disorders, has been widely touted, of late, as effective in decreasing the incidence and severity of migraines. It is said to be useful as a preventive measure, but not to control the pain of an acute attack. Propanolol is something of a fad at the moment; its benefits are overrated and its side effects—insomnia, depression, vomiting, diarrhea, skin rashes, nightmares, fatigue— make it an undesirable treatment for migraines. Type 1 persons should especially avoid propanolol, as it can aggravate respiratory symptoms and possibly be fatal to asthmatics.

If a headache drug must be used, ergotamines (Cafergot is one) constrict blood vessels and can usually control a migraine if taken at the first twinge, although some say that aspirin does as well. The problem with any drug is that it can lead to dependence and lack of motivation to look for the cause of the disorder.

The best treatment for headaches is prevention: a lifestyle that is custom-tailored to exclude foods or substances to which you're allergic; moderation in activities; a regular health routine including clean air, exercise, and adequate rest; and an active campaign against worry and tension.

Intravenous Sodium Bicarbonate. Clinical ecologists are equipped to give intravenous sodium bicarbonate to treat dire Type 2 reactions. These alkali salts are safe and effective, but as yet are not widely available in this form for this purpose.

In general, Type 2 persons can take encouragement from the fact that more and more people are beginning to know and care about chemical allergies, that researchers are continually looking for new ways to effect relief, and that many physicians are now recognizing and diagnosing these formerly "incurable" symptoms. There's even a name and a category for the people who seem to suffer most.

THE UNIVERSAL REACTOR

A very small number—about 1 percent—of Type 2 patients are not fortunate enough to gain early diagnosis or treatment of their symptoms and go on to become universal reactors; that is, their immune systems become so run down that they react to everything.

Tom Brighton is a good example. He endured all the usual childhood diseases as well as Type 1 inhalant allergies to dust, pollens, and pets and a Type 2 intolerance to many odors and foods. At the age of 15 he got a summer job as busboy in the closely enclosed cafeteria of a new office building. The combination of cooking smells and chemical fumes from the walls and furnishings made him feel nauseated, dizzy, and confused, and he was unable to continue working there.

A job delivering newspapers proved equally debilitating, although he didn't know why, since the work was outdoors. But the newsprint was fresh and pungent, the area was heavy in industrial fumes and pollution, and once again he found himself too sick to work. His doctor diagnosed emotional stress and suggested psychiatric treatment. The psychiatrist found him "anxious and paranoid" and sent him home with heavy sedation.

Tom's health continued to decline. He contracted infectious hepatitis, which confined him to bed for several months. Migraine headaches began appearing with increasing frequency. The day his mother sprayed the bedroom with insecticide, Tom's toxin-burdened system rebelled and he was rushed to the hospital with convulsive seizures. Fortunately, a doctor there, recognizing that he might be allergic rather than psychotic, treated him accordingly and took him off all food and medication except for light intravenous nutrients.

As soon as Tom could walk again, the doctor sent him to an ecology unit, a small hospital devoted to allergy research and testing. Tom found he was allergic to practically everything. Life at home had to be completely reordered.

The phenols in plastic bother him, so he now uses a speaker phone to call the farm that grows the pesticide-free carrots he eats on a glass plate. He serves himself with a stainless-steel fork that's been washed with spring water and dried with cotton toweling. He writes away for exotic foods such as llama, mountain lion, whale, squirrel, and lotus root, which he eats in rotation, every four days, because they're foods he's never eaten before and thus he hasn't built up an intolerance to them.

Wherever he goes, he carries an emergency kit that contains injectable adrenalin in case of anaphylactic shock, antihistamines, bicarbonate of soda tablets, and a battery of food antigens. His body apparently has been accumulating toxins for years. The hepatitis weakened his immune system, the insecticide pushed him over the edge, and he suddenly became sensitive to the whole spectrum of foods, inhalants, and chemicals—a condition that qualified him for the unfortunate label of universal reactor.

Today Tom is a much improved and very cautious Type 2. He knows what he can and can't do, watches his diet meticulously, and limits his activities and social life to nontoxic persons and conditions. If you met Tom Brighton walking down the street, you would think he was a normal, neatly dressed, quiet, pleasant young man. One of the main reasons for his improvement was a special small hospital that knew exactly how to treat him.

THE ECOLOGY UNIT

Most universal reactors are too ill to be tested in an office. They react to everything: the plastic syringe that squirts the test antigen as well as the extract itself, traces of detergent used to wash the technician's jacket, the ink on the instruction sheet, the polish on another patient's shoes. There is no way to detect the universal reactor's many specific allergies, even in the well-controlled environment of a clinical ecologist's testing room.

The only alternative is the ecology unit, or environmental control unit, which differs from the ecology center mentioned earlier in the book. Ecology centers are not necessarily staffed with medical doctors, treat many different types of ailments, and have only outpatient facilities. In contrast, the ecology unit is a medically controlled hospital, staffed and run by M.D.s and D.O.s (Doctors of Osteopathy), most of whom have been certified by the American Board of Allergy and Immunology and who are also clinical ecologists. They cater to extremely allergic persons who stay for several weeks.

The ecology unit has one main purpose: to relieve the patient of exposure to edible, airborne, and contact substances that cause allergies and then to reintroduce them to him, one by one, while measuring his reactions. If only to confirm patients' suspicions that they are severely allergic rather than neurotic, psychotic, or hypochondriacal, ecology units provide a great service for universal reactors. Doctors who run these hospitals say that the percentage of patients sensitive to chemicals rises dramatically each year as the quality of the environment—because of increased pollution—goes down.

Ecology units are not inexpensive. A three-week stay can cost $10,000 or more, and health insurers, still under the yoke of traditional medicine, may question the need for such costly "diagnostic tests." But expense is not the major problem. The real test is returning to your old environment and applying what you've learned.

At present there are ecology units in Colorado, Connecticut, Illinois, North Carolina, and Texas, and more keep springing up across the country. Many have a six-month waiting list. Their program is rigid. You, the patient, move into a bare cell of a room where all the variables are controlled—the air you breathe as well as everything you touch, smell, eat, and drink.

Television sets are glass-enclosed and special glass reading boxes are available to shield you from the newsprint fumes of books and magazines. Wooden games are supplied, but no playing cards or typewriters. Your wardrobe is limited to cotton garments that have never been dry-cleaned with chemicals or washed in strong-smelling detergent. You may have guests from the outside only if they're willing to be "purified" of possible fumes or pollutants. .

The first step in treatment is a fast, eliminating all solids and liquids except spring water. This can be a trying few days if you're withdrawing from food addiction, as many patients are. By the fourth day you may suddenly start to feel better. This gives you the spurt of encouragement to continue. After about five days pure, organic, unseasoned foods are added one by one. You're taught how to look for and record all reactions. Gradually, you're taken to a separate room and exposed to chemicals. Detailed testing continues until you have a good idea of your many sensitivities. Armed with this knowledge, you're once again returned to the real world, where you learn to assimilate this knowledge into a new style of living.

California's Dr. Phyllis Saifer is known to both patients and colleagues as a pioneer clinical ecologist and one of the movement's most articulate spokespersons. She is also a universal reactor. Before she realized what was making her ill, she consulted many doctors, including two psychiatrists who insisted she was suffering from stress and a "deprived childhood." Since she was a woman in a "man's field," they felt it was quite understandable that she would have emotional problems severe enough to cause physical symptoms.

In 1978, at a Society for Clinical Ecology meeting, she met Dr. Bill Rea, a vascular surgeon and head of the environmental unit in Dallas, Texas. As Dr. Saifer reports: "My health had continued to deteriorate so that symptoms of fatigue, depression, muscle aching, nasal congestion, generalized itching and bloating, anxiety, photophobia (light sensitivity), irritability, headache, chills, and so forth had become a daily phenomenon. I was at the point of thinking that I would have to stop working. I'd been taking a history on a patient and looked down half an hour later to find that I'd written nothing.

"I was nearly desperate to know what was going on in my body. Even if I had cancer at least I'd know what I had and what to do about it. When I met Bill Rea, I decided that I could no longer afford to put off the diagnostic and therapeutic visit to an ecology unit for the recommended three-week workup.

"I went to Dallas and entered the unit sick, depressed, frightened about the impending ordeal, and quite certain that it would be impossible to maintain a strictly disciplined regimen when I came home. As usual, I was anesthetized (mentally dulled) by the airport pollution and airplane fumes, and an exposure to perfume at the admissions desk left me crying for the next eighteen hours.

"In the controlled environment of the ecology unit, the nurses are in cotton uniforms and do not wear scent of any sort. The rooms are done with porcelain, aluminum, tile, and chemically untreated plasterboard. Beds and other furniture are steel and stripped (unvarnished) wood. Linens are all cotton, carefully washed in natural soap and rinsed with baking soda. Telephones are made of ceramic and the lighting is incandescent and glass."

Writing in a diary she kept of the experience, Dr. Saifer described a battery of challenges and reactions, starting with a fast. On the fourth day her withdrawal symptoms let up and she was able to test for chemicals. For the first time she began to realize how many of her "psychological" ailments were physical, caused by ordinary substances in the environment. The sadness of learning she was one of a tiny percentage of universally reactive patients was alleviated by the joy and relief of finally having a medical diagnosis with prospects of treatment and continued improvement.

It took three days for Dr. Saifer to recover from the effects of the airplane trip home, and she came back to a house her husband had stripped of vinyl, latex, plastic, and as many synthetic fibers as he could get rid of.

"The financial cost is great," she noted in her diary. "Dealing with chemical sensitivities in an age of plastic food, polluted air, and synthetic clothing is not within the means of many people. I also know I shall have to be a recluse for awhile and be terribly dependent on other people for shopping. Clothing stores, drugstores, and grocery stores are my enemies, and I'll have to do my work with my pair of 'dress jeans' and several cotton shirts.

"But it feels good. It's worth the effort, and I'm sure I won't miss the rest of the world one bit. The relief of having answers, and a therapeutic regimen that I know produces results, makes the task ahead a pleasurable challenge."

In March 1979 Dr. Saifer made a final entry: "It is sixteen months later and I really am better. If I do have an allergic reaction it's shorter and less severe. I've settled on one meal a day, dinner, because I found that all foods induce a mild fatigue and I can't afford to be drowsy in the office. My entire wardrobe is cotton and woolen, our bedding is cotton and wool, and I sleep on a rolled-up towel for a pillow. We use a microwave oven because the electric oven has some self-cleaning chemical on it that bothers me. Overall, I am feeling remarkably cheerful because all the hard work, deprivations, and restrictions have paid off."

Today she says, "I've continued to improve steadily, though it's five years later and I'm not 'cured.' Vitamins are now tolerable and seem to help certain symptoms. Transfer factor has been the greatest find; it keeps the T cells up and thus eliminates some of the prolonged reactions. Just with living carefully, improvement is constant. It almost suggests that many years' accumulation of toxins must slowly be leaving my body. Each year brings something new that helps a little bit."

It should be mentioned here that ecology units are not for everyone. Ninety-nine percent of Type 2 patients can do as well or better for their symptoms with proper medical care and changes of lifestyle. Yet for some people, like Tom Brighton and Phyllis Saifer, the ecology unit is a godsend. Its use is indicated in four instances for a patient: when he is having life-threatening reactions, when he lives too far from a clinical ecologist to be treated, when he has exceedingly complex and baffling symptoms, or when he is so confused by cerebral symptoms that he can't function.

If you fit any of those descriptions, be sure your doctor sends you to a recognized ecology unit. Anyone can call himself a clinical ecologist, so choose a hospital run by a doctor who is a certified member of the Society for Clinical Ecology. (See Chapter 5 for detailed information.)

The majority of universal reactors, because of lack of knowledge, ability, or patience, have not yet learned to take charge of their environments. Once they do, they can usually live as Type 2 persons who enjoy their families, many of the normal pleasures of life, and the benefits of good meals and healthy eating. Understanding food sensitivities is one of the prime factors in controlling both Type 1 and Type 2 allergies. The immediate beneficial effects of improving your diet may be a pleasant and unexpected bonus.

Chapter 4

ALL ABOUT FOODS

In March 1981 about 1,800 specialists attended the thirty-seventh annual meeting of the American Academy of Allergy at the Hilton Hotel in San Francisco, the largest such gathering ever held. Dr. Donald D. Stevenson of the Scripps Clinic and Research Foundation in La Jolla, California, told of a woman patient who took a few sips of wine and then went into anaphylactic shock, nearly suffocating. Months of medical sleuthing followed her attack but revealed nothing. Standard allergy tests, including a detailed food-elimination diet, gave no indication of sensitivities. Doctors were baffled.

Then one night at a friend's home, the woman again sipped some wine and the same thing happened. Within minutes, she was on her way to the hospital. When she recovered, she realized there had to be a difference between the wine she'd had at her friend's house and the wine she had drunk elsewhere, which gave her no problems.

Painstaking analysis finally revealed that the cork in her friend's wine had been treated with a food preservative called potassium metabisulfite, to which she was highly sensitive. Tiny fragments of cork floating in the wine had caused her reaction. When Dr. Stevenson presented his paper at the conference, he had the sensation that "light bulbs went on all over the audience" as his colleagues saw a possible explanation for some of their own patients' unsolved ailments.

Such experiences are happening everywhere, as both doctors and patients break away from conventional thinking and begin to realize how their diagnostic powers have been limited by man-made borders. Too many people still assсciate food allergy with traditional responses such as hives, headaches, and upset stomachs caused by traditionally offensive foods such as milk, citrus fruit, and eggs.

According to Dr. Marshall Mandell, these familiar and immediate (or slightly delayed) reactions account for only one-tenth of all food allergies. The other 90 percent are the vast range of symptoms from anemia to vertigo that people experience when they become sensitized to chemical additives such as metabisulfite, when they eat certain foods too frequently, when they eat unsuspected allergenic foods, or when they develop an addiction. Clinical ecologists believe that food allergies will one day be shown to be major offenders in many ailments whose causes are now unknown, including arthritis, cancer, and heart disease.

THE FOUR FOOD REACTIONS

The four patterns of allergic reactions to foods are *fixed, cumulative, variable, and addictive*. They all affect both Type 1 and Type 2 persons, but addiction is more common among the latter.

A *fixed* reaction is one that happens whenever a food is eaten. Every time you eat sugar you get a headache. Technically, that means that the allergens you've swallowed have met the trouble-causing sensitized cells right in your digestive tract. When it takes time for the allergens to travel through the bloodstream and encounter the sensitized cells in other body systems, you get a delayed fixed reaction. This can come half an hour to forty-eight hours later and can cause both Type 1 and Type 2 symptoms. Fixed reactions can be either mild or severe and can range from a few sniffles to anaphylactic shock, but the reaction is always the same.

A second type of food reaction is called *cumulative*, which means that allergens have to accumulate in your body before you react. They may do so over a certain period of time. Say you eat ten strawberries on Monday, ten more on Tuesday and ten more on Wednesday. You can tolerate ten or twenty strawberries but not thirty, and so on the third day you react. In most people, tiny food particles leak through the intestines and float around in the bloodstream for from four to seven days. As long as there is a trace of food in your body, eating more of the same food within the four-to-seven day period can cause an accumulation.

It can also happen immediately, however. Suppose you're a

Type 1 person who reacts to both strawberries and blooming acacia. If you eat strawberries in your kitchen with the windows
closed you may be fine. But if you take them into the garden to eat
under the acacia, the cumulative effect of the food plus the pollen
will push you over your tolerance threshold and give you symptoms. The same thing may happen with a Type 2 person who
might not be bothered by tobacco smoke until someone walks by
wearing strong perfume. Any two or more allergens can accumulate and cause a problem.

New evidence suggests that some substances—particularly
food and pollens—cross-react to cause both Type 1 and Type 2
symptoms; for instance, you may eat bread with no problems ten
months a year, but when certain grasses are pollinating you'll find
yourself unable to tolerate wheat because the grass pollens have
enhanced or triggered your allergy to wheat. If you're grass-sensi-
tive, a good rule to follow is to avoid wheat, bran, corn, barley,
oats, rye, rice and sugar cane—all members of the same biological
food family—as much as possible during grass season.

Then there's the *variable* response to foods, which also applies
to Types 1 and 2. In this case your reaction is unpredictable because
the symptoms are caused by a combination of factors. If you eat
chocolate on a smoggy day, you may get a headache. If you eat
chocolate after you have exercised vigorously and are perspiring,
your skin may break out. If you eat chocolate at the same time as
you eat wheat, you may get stomach cramps. It often takes a bit of
sleuthing to find out why the same food causes different symptoms.

The *addictive* reaction is remarkably similar to a drug addiction in that you become hooked on a particular food, need con-
tinual "fixes," and experience mild to severe withdrawal symptoms
when you can't get it. This is mainly a Type 2 symptom, although
Type 1 persons occasionally become food-addicted and usually
neither type knows what's happening. The reason is that traditional food allergies are supposed to give you headaches or nausea
and make you feel worse; when you're addicted, however, you
experience the opposite reaction: an instant lift from the food and a
momentary surge of well-being.

Here's a typical case. Jim wakes up every morning feeling
tired and grumpy. The moment he eats toast and cereal, his wheat
fix, he comes alive and feels wonderful. He limits himself to a
small vegetable salad for lunch, so by three in the afternoon he's

hungry for wheat. An ice cream cone gives him a spurt of energy. He assumes it comes from the sugar in the ice cream, when actually it's the wheat in the cone. No matter what he has for dinner, he doesn't feel satisfied unless he finishes with cake, cookies, or crackers and cheese.

The cycle starts again the next day. Jim's body is physiologically dependent on wheat. A number of hours after he eats it he feels depressed, irritable, angry at nothing—the beginning of the withdrawal stage—until he eats more wheat. Food addiction is a repeated cycle of getting a fix, experiencing the first pangs of withdrawal, and then taking another fix. If no fix is available, the person can experience such symptoms as chills and trembling, sweating, depression, headache, fever, waves of paranoia, and even vomiting and diarrhea, much like a drug addict's experience of cold-turkey withdrawal symptoms. This painful interval can last from one to four days.

A person can only become addicted, in the sense described here, to a food to which he is allergic; for example, at some period in his life, whether as a child or as an adult, Jim eats wheat and reacts. He might sneeze, cough, faint, feel either tense or lethargic, become bloated, or get a headache. Whatever the symptoms, his body is telling him that he's sensitive to that particular food. If he continues to eat wheat at meal after meal, day after day, his body will suppress the acute symptoms because of the constant exposure. The allergy then becomes "masked" and leads to a steady erosion of health, often manifesting itself in a chronic ailment such as colitis, arthritis, or depression.

If Jim stops eating wheat, his addicted body protests with unpleasant withdrawal symptoms. But if he continues to stay away from wheat, the withdrawal will end, his system will start to heal, his chronic disease will diminish or disappear, and he'll regain his health. The main difference between Jim and a drug addict is that Jim doesn't know he's hooked. Tell him he's allergic to wheat and he'll deny it vigorously because it's the only food that picks him up and makes him feel better. Ironically, the food that causes the problem is also the food that relieves the symptoms. Curing such an addiction is often easier than diagnosing it.

Idaho physician Thomas McDevitt believes that Prince Vlad Tepes, the fifteenth-century Transylvanian model for the fictional vampire Dracula, was allergy-addicted to human blood and became violent only when he started to feel withdrawal symptoms. If doctors had known then what they know now, perhaps Prince Tepes would have been broken of his addiction and Dracula might never have gained immortality in the horror Hall of Fame.

At the end of Chapter 1 there are several questions about eating habits. The first one asked if you have ever felt a strong craving for a particular food. If you answered yes, you may be addicted to that food. Positive replies to questions 2, 3, and 4— indicating that you sometimes feel you would go anywhere or pay anything for a certain food; that you feel weak, irritable, and frustrated until you get it; and that your symptoms disappear the moment you eat it—are further signs of possible food addiction. The fifth question, asking if you can sometimes eat and eat and yet not feel full, is a strong clue that food allergies may be affecting your appestat, the appetite control center in your brain. This malfunctioning of the appestat is a direct contributing factor to obesity, about which we will have more to say.

The cost of food allergy-addiction is heavy in many ways. Like the heroin addict, you can begin to get hooked on your own fixes, wanting more and more of them. If you're tied to chocolate, for instance, eating it stops your withdrawal symptoms of feeling weary and irritable and seems to give you instant energy. You want that energy often during your busy day, and your bathroom scale will soon begin to show it.

Even more important is the fact that food allergy-addictions do not stand still. Like a love affair, they either flourish or fade. Improvement comes only with not eating the food, and since many people have no idea what they're allergic to, the problem usually gets worse. The initial symptoms disappear and become masked, only to reappear eventually as a more severe and possibly devastating illness. Thus there are many reasons besides obesity why a food addiction is unhealthy. The key to controlling all these symptoms lies in a regulated scheme of eating.

THE FOOD SENSITIVITY DIETS

Now that you know about food reactions, we're going to offer you a choice of four allergy diets: The Basic Food Sensitivity Diet (FSD) is to rid your body of possibly allergenic foods and help you find out what you're allergic to. The Vegetarian FSD is the same thing for non-meat-eaters, and the Candida FSD is adapted for people who are mold-sensitive or who may have candidiasis. In the next section, the 5/5 Allergy-Obesity Diet (AOD) should take off five or more pounds in the first five days.

Before you start any one of these diets, talk it over with your doctor. If you're taking prescription medication be sure to keep taking it. Your physician may find that he can lower your doses of drugs or even completely eliminate them—particularly if they're antihistamines or antihypertensives—as you progress. Do, temporarily, stop taking vitamin pills, as most of them contain dyes, additives, and probably such allergenic foods as corn or yeast.

Don't start a diet if you're pregnant; if you smoke (unless you're willing to stop); if you're suffering an acute illness such as viral infection, cold, or flu; if you've recently undergone surgery or severe trauma; or during pollen season if you're a Type 1. It's important to be able to relate your symptoms to foods rather than to other causes.

Keep a careful journal of all foods you eat and how you feel, even several hours later or the next day. Write down everything, whether you think it's trivial or not. Your diary should look something like this:

DATE	WEIGHT	TIME	FOOD	REACTION
8/17	150	12:00 noon	Two bananas	None
		3:00 P.M.	Tomato, lettuce, tuna, lemon juice	
		3:15 P.M.		Mild headache
		6:00 P.M.	Broiled chicken, potato, peas	
		8:20 P.M.		Eye itch
8/18	148	7:00 A.M.		Feeling great

These next five rules may seem stringent but it will be worth your while to stick to them, at least for the seven days you're on the Basic FSD. If they seem very restrictive, you are eating too many of the wrong foods in your normal diet and you should change your patterns anyway. Allergic people need support and nutrition from their daily intake, not added stresses.

1. Avoid tap water in favor of bottled spring water, carbonated mineral water such as Perrier, or bottled fresh fruit or vegetable juice. Be sure to drink six or more glasses of fluid each day. For most people the offending elements in water are, in this order: chlorine, pesticides and other organic chemicals; and minerals such as fluoride, sulfur, copper, aluminum, and lead.

Distilling water removes minerals and salts but does not always remove all the chlorine or other chemicals, so if you're a chlorine-sensitive Type 2 be cautious with distilled water. Spring waters are usually free of chlorine only; where they come from determines whether they are pesticide-free and which minerals are present.

All liquids should be stored in and drunk from glass or ceramic containers as those made from soft plastic leach out components of plastic into the contents. If pure water is unavailable, boil tap water vigorously in an open pot for ten minutes, allow it to cool until no more steam comes off, and store it in glass bottles.

2. Avoid all processed foods, including anything that contains additives or preservatives or is packaged in plastic. Ideally, all fruits and vegetables should be free of pesticides and chemicals, but truly organic foods are often hard to find. Do not eat canned food, as you may react to the phenol lining of the can rather than its contents and thus reach the wrong conclusions.

Commercially frozen foods are not recommended because of the added sugars and the plastic packaging. Foods packaged in boxes, cellophane, or glass are fine if they meet the other requirements. Buy meats and fish from a butcher so that they're wrapped in paper instead of heat-sealed polyurethane and polystyrene. Home-frozen meats and other vegetables wrapped in foil are permitted, as are fresh fruits or vegetables home-preserved in jars without sugar. Dried fruits are acceptable if they are unsulfured and preservative-free, and so are fresh or dried herbs, although powdered herbs in jars often have anti-caking agents added to make them pour easily.

Be sure to cut all fat from meat, because that's where the pesticides accumulate. Do it before cooking so that the fat doesn't melt and become absorbed into the meat. Oils should be labeled cold pressed, cold processed, or expeller pressed, which means they've been squeezed from nuts and seeds by a mechanical process that doesn't use chemicals. Oils not so labeled are likely to have been extracted by the use of the solvent hexane.

3. Try to eat a wide variety of foods, including ones not usually on your menu. If you haven't eaten something before, you probably haven't had a chance to become sensitive to it. Rotate your foods so that if you eat one thing the first day, you wait at least three days before eating it again. This will break food-addiction patterns and keep new ones from forming.

4. Be wary of restaurants. A common practice to prevent discoloration is to dip fresh fruit and vegetables in a solution of "potato whitener," or potassium metabisulfite, the additive found in the wine cork mentioned at the start of this chapter.

There are two excellent reasons not to "sulfite" foods. First, it can be very dangerous. Doctors at the Scripps Institute estimate that half a million asthma sufferers are sulfite-sensitive. Second, it is deceptive. Using sulfite for cosmetic purposes means that you could be eating a slice of "fresh" apple that is three weeks old. Some chefs just keep dunking and dunking.

In July 1982 the FDA declared sulfiting agents to be safe and acceptable for use. In February 1983 a "60 Minutes" television report called attention to the dangers of this practice, and a month later, the FDA issued a new regulation requiring retail food establishments that use sulfiting agents to so inform consumers by statements on menus, or to cease using them.

5. If you must go off the Basic FSD, be careful. Avoiding certain foods for several days may make you hypersensitive, and you may react much more strongly when you eat the foods again. If you know in advance that you'll be in a situation where you might stray,. try to fast twelve hours before and after eating the offending meal. When the immune system doesn't have to cope with other foods, it can give all its attention to dispatching the enemy.

You may feel worse the first three to five days on the diet as your body withdraws from foods to which you're accustomed. During this time, make a particular effort to eat as many new foods as you can. It will be normal to be hungry for or even to yearn for certain dishes, but it will be significant only if you actually crave a food. Note all reactions in your diary.

The Basic FSD, with its insistence on avoiding chemicals and processed foods, may seem heavily slanted toward Type 2 persons, but the diet is engineered for Type 1 persons as well, in the conviction that both types will benefit from eating "cleaner" foods in the same way that we all benefit from breathing cleaner air. Besides being recommended for both Type 1 and Type 2 persons, the Basic FSD should be followed by all people who suspect they may be mildly or markedly allergic.

The Basic Food Sensitivity Diet

The bill of fare for this diet features fresh, unprocessed meat, poultry, seafood, fruit, and vegetables. You might say that it's the way our primeval ancestors ate, before allergies—as we know them—became so prevalent. On this diet, simplicity does not mean lack of variety. For those who are used to eating similar foods every day, the challenge of eating an array of different foods may even spark culinary creativity.

The Basic FSD has two purposes. One is therapeutic: to clear your body of commonly allergenic foods to which you may be sensitive. Even if you prove not to be, the fact that you stop eating hotdogs and cupcakes and start eating wholesome, chemical-free foods will make you feel better.

The second purpose is diagnostic: to evaluate your responses to various foods, to keep careful notes, and eventually to develop a diet that limits or excludes the offending foods. The diet should be followed for seven days, and you should remember to record everything in your journal. Here's what you do:

1. *Eat fresh fruit, vegetables, meat, poultry, and seafood.*

2. *Do not eat sugar, cow's milk, wheat, eggs, corn, soy, yeast, caffeine, alcohol, or any products containing them.* These foods are the most common offenders. (For detailed lists, see Days 5, 8, 15, 22, 29, and 36 of the Allergy-Obesity Diet later in this chapter.)

3. *Avoid your favorite foods,* even if they're not on the taboo list. Anything that you eat daily, such as orange juice or tuna fish, should be put aside. People can become allergic to foods because of too frequent consumption.

The permitted foods are on two lists. You may add to either list anything that is fresh, unprocessed, and not in Rule 2. Eggs or corn, for instance, could not be included even though they might be fresh and unprocessed.

The idea is to eat as many *different* foods as possible spaced as far apart as possible. If you're the least bit creative, you'll find there are more than enough choices for a variety in menus. Each day try to choose at least one food from each group: protein, vegetables, starch, fruit, fat, and nuts and seeds. Sweeteners and seasonings are optional. Proceed this way:

Day 1: Any foods from List A

Day 2: Any foods from List B

Day 3: Any foods from List A not eaten on Day 1

Day 4: Any foods from List B not eaten on Day 2

Day 5: Any foods from List A not eaten on Day 3

Day 6: Any foods from List B not eaten on Day 4

Day 7: Any foods from List A

Days 5 and 6 *can* include foods from Days 1 and 2, but if you're able to avoid them, so much the better. Foods separated by a slash (lemon/lime) are in the same biological family and, if possible, should be eaten at least two days apart. Try to prepare all your meals at home from fresh, natural, ingredients.

LIST A

Protein

Mollusks: abalone/snail/squid/mussels/oysters/scallops
Crustaceans: crab/crayfish/lobster/prawn/shrimp
Duck/goose
Frog/turtle

Deer
Beef/veal/lamb/goat/buffalo

Vegetables

Asparagus/chives/garlic/leek/onions/shallots
Beets/chard/spinach
Alfalfa sprouts/all beans/peas/jicama/lentils/peanuts
Cucumber/squashes
Dandelion greens/endive/artichoke/lettuce/chicory
Okra

Starch

Barley/millet/oat/rice/rye/wild rice

Fruit

Avocado
Coconut/dates
Pineapple
Bananas/plantains
Figs
Grapefruit/kumquats/lemons/limes/oranges/tangelos/tangerines
Papaya
Passion fruit
Pomegranates
Guava
Persimmons
Melon/pumpkin

Sweeteners

Date sugar
Honey—clover, star thistle, orange blossom

Fat (cold pressed oil)

Avocado oil
Walnut oil
Safflower oil

Sunflower oil
Pumpkin seed oil

Seasonings

Cardamom/ginger/turmeric
Vanilla bean
Nutmeg
Cinnamon/bay leaf
Fenugreek
Allspice
Clove
Tarragon

Nuts and Seeds

Walnuts/pecans
Chestnuts
Brazil nuts
Pumpkin seeds
Sunflower seeds

LIST B

Protein

All fish that don't have shells
Dove/pigeon
Partridge
Chicken/pheasant/quail
Rabbit
Whale
Pork
Turkey

Vegetables

Rhubarb
Broccoli/Brussels sprouts/cabbage/cauliflower/Chinese cabbage/col-
    lards/kale/kohlrabi/mustard greens/radishes/rutabagas/turnips/
    watercress
Carrots/peppers/tomatoes

Starch

Yams
Buckwheat
Potatoes
Sweet potatoes

Fruit

Currants
Apples/loquats/pears/quince/apricots/cherries/peaches/nectarines/
   plums/prunes
Mango
Grapes/raisins
Kiwi fruit
Cranberries/blueberries
All other berries

Sweeteners

Maple sugar or syrup
Honey—sage, rosemary

Fat (cold pressed oil)

Olive oil
Apricot kernel oil
Hazelnut oil
Sesame oil
Cottonseed oil

Seasonings

Black pepper
Mustard seed
Poppyseed
Cumin/anise/caraway/chervil/coriander/dill/basil/marjoram/orega-
   no/sage/thyme/mint

Nuts and Seeds

Filberts
Almonds
Cashews/pistachios (not red-dyed)
Sesame seeds

Once you're into the Basic FSD, other questions may occur to you, such as the use of table salt. Since it commonly contains dextrose (corn sugar) and sodium aluminum silicate as anticaking agents, it should be avoided, but you may use sea salt (you may have to grind your own). Many people who react adversely to additives and impurities in table salt are not allergic to pure sodium chloride.

A variety of ingredients will enhance the flavors of your dishes; the most popular natural seasonings are lemon juice, vinegar, ginger, garlic, and onions. Herbs and spices should be fresh or dried whole and ground at home. Supermarkets now have special shelves devoted to salt-free foods and are continually introducing new products.

The Basic FSD is not a weight-reduction diet, but you may be cutting 20 percent or more of your caloric intake by removing meat fats, milk and milk products, and most cereal grains. Keep track of your weight. If you want to lose weight, fine. If not, replace that caloric loss by increasing your intake of the allowed foods.

Here are four days of sample menus to start you on the Basic FSD. Recipes follow for dishes marked with an asterisk (*).

DAY 1

Breakfast: Bananas
           Filberts
Lunch: Spinach salad with lemon pepper dressing *
Dinner: Duck with ginger orange glaze*
           Roasted yams*
           Sesame broccoli*

DAY 2

Breakfast: Hot oatmeal with dates and coconut
Lunch: Roquefort walnut salad*
Dinner: Broiled lamb chops
           Millet dressing with currants*
           Steamed zucchini
           Apples

DAY 3

Breakfast: Hot whole buckwheat with maple syrup
Lunch: Cabbage cauliflower salad with raisins*
Dinner: Sautéed chicken with lime*
           Baked potatoes
           Steamed Brussels sprouts
           Spearmint snow*

DAY 4

Breakfast: Hot barley with pecans and figs
Lunch: Lentil soup*
           Rye crackers
Dinner: Crispy fish*
           Brown rice
           Steamed yellow squash
           Honey apricot ice*

Recipes

These recipes all serve two to four persons and should provide some ideas for simple, nutritious, nonallergenic meals during the week of your Basic Food Sensitivity Diet.

Spinach Salad with Lemon Pepper Dressing

1 bunch fresh spinach
1 tomato, sliced
1 green pepper, sliced
1 avocado, sliced
3 tablespoons apricot kernel oil
6 teaspoons lemon juice
½ teaspoon freshly ground black pepper
½ teaspoon dried oregano

Wash spinach thoroughly, cut off stems, tear into bite-size pieces, and place in a large salad bowl. Add tomato, green pepper, and avocado. Mix oil, lemon juice, black pepper, and oregano and pour over vegetables just before serving.

Duck with Ginger Orange Glaze

1¾ lb. duck
1 tablespoon sesame oil
¼ cup orange juice
2 tablespoons fresh ginger, finely chopped
(Note: This recipe is for a fresh duck. If frozen duck is used, follow package instructions.) Preheat oven to 375 degrees. Place duck with breast side down on roasting pan; bake for 30 minutes. Combine oil, orange juice, and ginger in a saucepan and simmer gently to make glaze. After 30 minutes, turn duck over, glaze exposed side, and bake for 30 minutes more. Turn duck again, glaze top, turn up the oven to 450 degrees, and roast for another 15 minutes, watching carefully to make sure duck doesn't burn.

Variations: This recipe is also good with chicken. Depending on your rotation, glazes could be made from any combination of oils, ginger, garlic, lemons, oranges, limes, tangerines, and honeys.

Roasted Yams (to go with duck)

Peel and cut 3 medium-size yams into approximately 2-inch chunks. Place in a lightly oiled roasting pan underneath the duck and place the duck on a rack on top of them. During cooking, the yams will absorb juice from both the duck and the ginger orange glaze. By the time the duck is done, the yams will be cooked and the glaze should begin to carmelize. If it hasn't carmelized, remove the duck, turn up the oven to 450 degrees, and continue baking for 5 to 10 more minutes while preparing the duck for serving.

Sesame Broccoli

1 average bunch broccoli
⅛ cup sesame seeds
Sesame oil to cover pan
Roasted sesame oil (optional but good; available in health food
  stores)
Wash broccoli, cut off stems, and split into flowerets. Heat oil and brown sesame seeds for 1 to 2 minutes. Remove from pan and

sauté broccoli for about five minutes. Broccoli will still be crunchy when done. Add sesame seeds and a few drops of roasted sesame oil if desired.

Roquefort Walnut Salad

1 medium head romaine lettuce
¼ cup coarsely chopped walnuts
1 cucumber, sliced
½ cup crumbled Roquefort cheese (made from sheep's milk)
2 tablespoons walnut oil
3 tablespoons apple juice

Wash lettuce thoroughly, tear into bite-size pieces, and place in a large salad bowl. Add walnuts, cucumber, and cheese. Mix together oil and apple juice and pour over vegetables.

Variation: If your rotation allows, you can also add freshly ground black pepper and very thin slices of red onion.

Millet Dressing with Currants

2 cups water
1 cup dry millet
2 tablespoons walnut oil
½ large head garlic, chopped
3 stalks celery (with tops), chopped
½ cup currants

Add millet to boiling water and cook over medium heat for 30 minutes or until done. Sauté garlic and celery in oil, then add cooked millet and currants. Bake uncovered for 20 minutes at 350 degrees.

Cabbage Cauliflower Salad with Raisins

1 small head red cabbage
1 small head green cabbage
1 medium cauliflower
1 cup raisins
6 tablespoons avocado oil
8 tablespoons grapefruit juice

Slice cabbages into ¼ inch strips and cut cauliflower into small flowerets. Steam vegetables together or separately for 2 minutes, then plunge immediately into ice water to stop the cooking process so that vegetables don't become soggy. Combine all ingredients and chill for 1 hour before serving.

Sautéed Chicken with Limes

1 medium frying chicken (cut up) or the equivalent in chicken
   parts
Olive oil
4 teaspoons dried sweet basil
2 limes

Cover the bottom of a large heated skillet generously with oil (a whole chicken may require two skillets). Cook chicken over medium heat for 10 to 15 minutes or until golden brown. Turn chicken over, place a lime slice on each piece, and squeeze juice from remaining lime over the top. Sprinkle generously with sweet basil, crushing the leaves between your fingers. Continue cooking for another 10 to 15 minutes. If you turn pieces again, keep the lime slice on top.

Spearmint Snow

3 cups boiling water
6 heaping teaspoons spearmint tea (or 6 teabags)
2 heaping tablespoons honey

Steep tea in water for 20 minutes, then strain to remove leaves. Stir in honey until it is completely dissolved. Freeze in a glass or metal bowl for 4 to 6 hours (time will vary according to freezer temperature), stirring every half hour to break up ice crystals until they resemble snow. If you overfreeze, crack ice into large chunks with a roasting fork and crush in a food processor for a few seconds before serving.

   Variations: This can be made with any kind of tea and any type of honey.

Lentil Soup

1½ cups dry lentils
4½ cups pure water
3 medium carrots, peeled and chopped
¼ cup coarsely chopped parsley
¾ teaspoon celery seeds

Combine all ingredients in a large pot, cover, and bake at 350 degrees or cook over medium heat for 1½ hours. For a thicker soup, continue to cook another half hour.

Crispy Fish

4 small fish filets
2 small onions
¾ cup rice flour
¼ cup tapioca flour
Safflower oil

Combine flours in a paper bag and coat fish by shaking it gently in the mixture. Cover the bottom of a large heated skillet generously with oil and add fish. Cook over medium heat until each side is browned. Slice onions in very thin rings and simmer in pan around the edges of the fish.

Variation: This can be made with any combination of flours and with added herbs and spices. Use 4 teaspoons of seasoning per cup of flour. This is also excellent for frying chicken and for breading meats and vegetables.

Honey Apricot Ice

1 quart unsweetened apricot juice or nectar
6 ounces dried apricots (unsulfured)
2 heaping tablespoons honey

Stew apricots for 20 minutes in apricot juice, add honey and stir until melted, then let sit until cool. Purée in blender or food processor until smooth. Freeze, stirring occasionally, for several hours.

The Vegetarian Food Sensitivity Diet

There are two variations to the Basic FSD that may better suit your needs. One is vegetarian or semivegetarian and excludes red meat. This diet suggests certain combinations such as lentils and rice or kidney beans and sesame seeds that can provide more protein than a steak, but they have to be eaten together. Vegetables, fruits, starches, sweeteners, fats, seasonings, and nuts and seeds are the same on the Vegetarian FSD as they are on the Basic FSD. Substitute the following foods for the proteins listed on the Basic FSD.

LIST A

Protein

If you eat fish, include:
   Mollusks: abalone/snails/squid/mussels/oysters/scallops
   Crustaceans: crab/crayfish/lobster/prawn/shrimp
   Frog/turtle
If you eat fowl, you may also include:
   Duck/goose
   Chicken/pheasant/quail
   Turkey
Replace meat with
   Almonds with buckwheat
   Cashews with buckwheat

LIST B

Protein

If you eat fish, include:
   All fish that swim
   Whale
If you eat fowl, you may also include:
   Dove/pigeon
   Partridge
Replace meat with any of the following, combined with beans and
      lentils:
   Barley
   Millet
   Sesame seeds

Brazil nuts
Rye

The Candida Food Sensitivity Diet

This diet is for people who are extremely mold-sensitive or who suspect, because of a history of recurrent monilia or other symptoms, that they may have candidiasis. In addition to the Basic FSD, add these rules:

Omit dried fruits, dried herbs, and herb teas.
Omit all nuts and seeds and their products.
Omit fruit juices unless home-squeezed.
Omit all spices.
Omit mushrooms, truffles, and all mold foods.

In extreme cases, you may want to exclude beef and all products from animals fed mold-derived antibiotics such as penicillin. Organic meats are available at some health-food stores, or see "Where to Send for Products" for mail-order sources.

The rest of the Candida FSD is the same as the Basic FSD, with an emphasis on avoiding vitamins (many are derived from yeast, such as B and B complex) and eliminating baked goods made with yeast, all kinds of cheese, fermented beverages, and vinegar. These are already excluded from the Basic FSD but the list is repeated here for emphasis.

Any food that shows traces of mold should immediately be discarded, of course, and since all the things you're eating are relatively free of preservatives, mold growth will be more of a problem than it is ordinarily. One woman on the Candida diet who loved to eat persimmons unexpectedly had a strong reaction to the fruit. She discovered that the sweet, juicy persimmons had become overripe and had started to ferment and produce mold, which caused her troubling symptoms. Refrigerate as much as you can, including starches.

CHALLENGE YOURSELF

Afer seven days on any of the FSDs, you're ready to start challenge testing for the foods you've been avoiding, or for any you've been eating that seemed to cause symptoms. You should have a master list of all tolerated foods, offending foods, and those you question. Avoid the foods that you know cause problems and test the questionable ones.

Here's what to do: Eat only the food being tested at a particular meal. If it's corn, for example, your meal should consist of corn on the cob or cornmeal mush cooked in pure water. *No other food or condiments can be eaten at the same meal.*

Take your pulse before ingestion and at ten-minute intervals afterward for the first hour. Note any rise in pulse rate. If you have symptoms, an antihistamine or some alkali salts, and up to three grams (3,000 units) of vitamin C should help. Persistent symptoms may require four tablespoons of milk of magnesia in a pint of water, or up to ten grams of vitamin C (if you tolerate it) for a laxative effect. It is wise to eliminate the offending food from your body as quickly as possible.

If you have a history of extreme reactions, or the least suspicion that you may be supersensitive to a food, don't take chances. Leave that test for a professional. You might also have self-injectable adrenalin available in case of a severe reaction to a food you hadn't suspected. Get a prescription for the EpiPen Auto-Injector from your doctor.

When you have no response to a test substance, wait forty-eight hours to be sure you don't experience delayed symptoms. Stay on the Basic FSD, and then start testing again. Exclude from your diet the food you have already tested, even though you had no response to it, as it could react with another "nonoffending" food and cause a cumulative reaction. Wait until you finish testing and your total allergic picture takes shape.

Your symptoms may also come from sources other than food, including the environment, emotional stresses, or unconscious suggestion. The only way to be certain it's a food is to retest in different conditions. After any reaction, wait five days before testing a new food, and at least a month before trying the food in question. By that time your diet will be more stabilized and your responses will be easier to assess.

As you continue to follow the Basic FSD, Vegetarian FSD, or Candida FSD and to challenge yourself with different foods, you will gradually get an overall picture of what you can eat with no problems, what you respond to slightly, and what you should avoid. If you reacted to no more than half the foods challenged, you have the potential of becoming a universal reactor and must immediately begin a strict rotary diet to prevent further sensitization.

Your diet will be as individual and "custom-tailored" to you as your wardrobe. Debbie Dadd can't eat beef, wheat, or fish, but feels splendid on a regime of fruits, vegetables, chicken, duck, turkey, eggs, cheese, and nuts. She can now even tolerate very small amounts of sugar and chocolate, which she shouldn't eat but occasionally does—and has no reaction.

This illustrates one happy aspect of allergy diets: after avoiding an offender for an appropriate period of time, usually eighteen months to two years, you can often begin to tolerate small amounts of the food at occasional intervals. But approach and try it with great caution.

The results of the Basic FSD and subsequent challenge testing should help you form a lasting pattern based on four rules:

1. Eat simpler meals.
2. Eat a large variety of foods. You mainly develop allergies to things you eat repeatedly.
3. Space your foods as far apart as possible. Whatever you eat on Monday, don't repeat until Wednesday or Thursday.
4. Once you find your "safe" path, stick to it. Don't slip into old habits, even if you think you're nonreactive to certain foods. When you know what foods you tolerate better than others, you'll find that you can go off your diet now and then, on special occasions, without paying a high price.

The more you eat sensible, nutritious meals, the more you'll build up a healthy body with a high tolerance level and the ability to resist other allergens in the environment. You won't make them disappear, but you can do your best to fight back, particularly when you're dealing with two of the greatest health problems of modern society.

ALCOHOLISM, OBESITY, AND THE 5/5 ALLERGY-OBESITY DIET

It is estimated that as many as 60 percent of the people who suffer from alcoholism or obesity have Type 2 addictive food allergies that either cause or aggravate their condition. If these persons make appropriate changes in diet and stick to them, their symptoms will disappear.

Alcoholism

The traditional view of an alcoholic is a person who is weak-willed, feels inferior and insecure, and has some sort of mental problem. Within the last decade, people have become aware of other possibilities. Dr. Theron Randolph did a series of tests and found that most of his alcoholic patients had no desire to drink ethyl alcohol in pure form, yet they craved alcoholic beverages that contained other ingredients. He gathered enough evidence to conclude that it was mainly the *foods* such as yeast, wheat, and sugar in these drinks—not the alcohol—to which they were addicted.

Two cases illustrate this phenomenon. The first deals with a 14-year-old boy interviewed on national television who told of how he started drinking beer one night at a party. It made him feel nauseated and sick, but he didn't want to admit this to his friends. After a while, he found he could tolerate the beer, began drinking it regularly, and soon noticed that he felt very bad when he stopped drinking it, even for a day. As soon as he gave in to his craving and took another glass, he felt fine again.

His worried parents took him to a physician who tested him for food allergies. The boy turned out to be highly sensitive to yeast. His need for beer was actually an allergic addiction to the yeast in the brew, not to the alcohol. Avoiding all forms of yeast soon curbed his "alcoholism."

The second case concerns a 32-year-old singer named Connie, who had a long history of this disease. Both her parents had Type 2 allergies, so severe, in fact, that they had to move from the polluted city air to a development near the ocean. It never occurred to them that Connie's drinking problem might be allergy-related until she came to stay with them after "drying out" in a sanitarium.

Sharing her parents' corn-free diet was disastrous, and triggered a new and intense craving for bourbon. Connie's mother rushed her to the allergist's office, where tests provoked a violent response to corn. Even though Connie had had no liquor in the hospital, she had been able to maintain her addiction by eating corn in foods. When deprived of all corn products, she experienced the strong withdrawal symptoms that showed she was addicted to the corn in bourbon, not to the alcohol.

Her sensitivity turned out to be so extreme that she must not only avoid the obvious forms of corn but also the myriad products in which it appears, such as catsup, candy, and foods made with cornstarch, corn syrup, corn sugar, corn oil, corn meal, corn flour, and so forth. She can't even lick stamps (the glue contains corn), drink from paper cups (coated with a corn product), use toothpaste, or take aspirin or most vitamin pills. Her addiction to wheat, a member of the same food family, is less acute but strong enough to warrant avoidance of wheat products as well.

The main benefit of the strict diet she now follows is that she no longer craves alcohol. The slightest lapse in diet, however, would give her an immediate corn or wheat "high" and trigger an acute craving for liquor that she would find almost impossible to resist. Many people find it just as hard to resist the foods themselves, and spend the greater part of their lives fighting the battle of the beltline.

Obesity

There are several reasons, besides all the obvious ones, for the allergic person not to carry extra weight:

It makes more work for the already taxed immune system.

It strains the breathing apparatus, which aggravates Type 1 respiratory symptoms. Dr. Constantine Falliers, an allergist in Denver, Colorado, says, "For a person with asthma or any kind of breathing problem, being overweight is like wearing a very tight garment. You don't have enough room for your muscles to expand in the lungs."

It stores chemicals. The more fat you have, the more you retain chemicals that constantly leach into your blood and can intensify Type 2 symptoms. Some Type 2 persons become discouraged when they first start to lose weight because they continue to have food cravings even though they're careful to avoid allergens. The problem comes from within. Dissolving fat releases chemicals into their bodies and causes abnormal hunger. When there's no more fat to melt, there are no more cravings.

Being underweight is not desirable, either, as you need reserves in case of accident or illness. Here's how to determine what your ideal weight should be:

For Men: Take 106 pounds for the first five feet and then add six pounds an inch. If you're 5-foot-11, that would be 106 plus 66 (6×11) = 172. A large-boned man can add 10 percent to make 189 pounds, and a man with a small frame should subtract 10 percent to arrive at 155.

For Women: Take 100 pounds for five feet of height and then add five pounds an inch. If you're 5-foot-5, you should weigh 125. A large-boned woman can add 10 percent to make 137.5 (125 plus 12.5 pounds, and a woman with a small frame should subtract 10 percent to make 112.5 (125 − 12.5) pounds.

There are four main ways that food allergies can stimulate weight gain: *addiction, cravings, appestat switch-off,* and *edema.* They all overlap and are mostly but not always Type 2 reactions. Let's take a look at each one.

Addiction. As explained earlier, many people are overweight because they're physiologically hooked on food. Usually it's a favorite dish—one they eat at least once a day—that supplies a fix, relieves their allergic symptoms, and gives them an instant lift. The food is generally something that tastes good, is fattening, such as chocolate or cheese (people rarely get hooked on celery), and insures continuing calories.

Cravings. All substances and conditions that cause allergies can cause acute hunger pangs, and that includes changes of weather, pills and medications, cooking odors, and tap water, to mention only a few. A craving can be for a specific food, such as a Tootsie Roll, or for a more general category, such as pasta.

A typical patient was a 28-year-old woman who had been overweight most of her life. She had tried a variety of fad diets and appetite suppressants, but couldn't break her compulsive need for sweets. She could control her eating in her own home. When someone brought ice cream, her favorite food, into the house, she would say, "Sorry, I can't have any. I'm on a diet." But when she was outside, exposed to traffic fumes, perfumes, and hairspray, she would rush to the nearest store and devour several scoops of mocha almond fudge.

The puzzle came together with the simple realization that chemical exposure caused an allergic reaction, which manifested itself in sudden, uncontrollable hunger. Tests showed a strong sensitivity to car exhaust, glycerin, and several other common environmental chemicals. As soon as she started avoiding these substances, her desire for sweets diminished and she was able to begin a sugar-free diet. Now that she knows her ice cream compulsion is an allergy, she controls her weight by getting away from the chemicals as fast as she can, and letting the desire subside.

Without depriving herself of anything, she tries to drive when traffic is light and to have products delivered to her home. She goes to a small beauty salon where the stylist knows her situation, and makes appointments on days when no one is getting a permanent or using hairspray. As long as she avoids the offending fumes, she has no problem with compulsive eating.

Sugar craving is quite common, especially among Type 2 persons, and has three specific sources: hormone imbalance, Candida sensitivity, or chemical exposure. One young woman who was twenty pounds overweight dated two men. When she dined with one she always felt embarrassed about her sweet tooth, and it became a joke between them. He'd tell the waiter, "Don't bother showing her the dessert cart. Just bring everything on it." Yet she could barely finish dinner, much less eat dessert, with the second man. Sublingual testing showed a strong sensitivity to smoke. The first chap was wedded to his pipe; the second never touched tobacco.

Once you suspect you may have this problem, you should be able to spot specific substances, foods or areas that seem to make you hungry. Like the lady who had to dash out of the beauty parlor for ice cream because she was sensitive to hairspray, you may find yourself craving cheddar cheese in the middle of sexual intercourse. It shouldn't take long for you to figure out that contraceptive foam (or some other synthetic chemical) is the culprit. Look for strong odors whenever you feel a craving.

Appestat Switch-Off. Scientists have learned that certain substances can go diretly to the brain and affect the appestat, or appetite control center, in the hypothalamus gland. When there are enough of these molecules to damage the appestat, it simply shuts down and refuses to fire off regulatory commands. Thus your brain gets no messages: no signal tells you that you've had enough to eat, you're full of food, and it's time to stop eating.

These reactions can be caused by anything—petting the dog, smelling a rose, scrambling eggs over a gas stove, or kissing a friend who's wearing cologne. Guests at cocktail parties sometimes find themselves grabbing hors d'oeuvres as fast as they can gulp them. It doesn't excuse bad manners, of course, but they could be feeling an allergic reaction to something as subtle as the corn in their bourbon.

If you never feel full or hungry after a meal, you may have an out-of-order appestat. Once you pinpoint the offending substance, you'll be able to reactivate your appestat by avoiding the allergen.

Edema. The latest available date show that edema, or fluid retention, is the most common form of allergic obesity. Edema is closely related to, and is often a result of, food addiction, and can account for five to twenty-five pounds of a person's weight in water bloat.

A 46-year-old man who had had a weight problem all his adult life went on diet after diet, but continued to be heavy. When he read an article on food allergies, he began to suspect his problem might be more than just "metabolism." He started monitoring his foods and noticed that he would gain three to five pounds the day after he ate cottage cheese. He decided to stop eating all milk products, and shed the bloat within forty-eight hours.

He kept up that regime for two months, substituting fresh meat, fruits, and vegetables for the dairy foods. Not only did he shrink a whole suit size, but he found that he could eat much more on his new diet without gaining an ounce. To test himself one day, he drank half a glass of milk, and within three hours he had severe stomach cramps, diarrhea, and a swollen midsection. Now he stays on his milk-free diet and maintains his slimmer figure even while he's consuming more calories.

Another example was a young nurse who had a favorite blue dress she could wear only after taking strong diuretics that allowed her to shed twelve pounds in three days. Challenge testing indicated reactions to apples, wheat, pork, and citrus fruit. She adjusted her diet to exclude those foods and found that she could maintain her blue-dress figure with no diuretics and only moderate calorie watching. You may have a similar problem; here's how to find out.

The 5/5 Allergy-Obesity Diet

The 5/5 AOD is so-called because overweight is often due to fluid retention. If your edema is allergic in origin, you will lose five (or more) pounds within five days; hence the term 5/5. The more allergic you are, the faster the weight will come off.

There's even an advantage to having allergic edema. Under normal conditions, there is absolutely no way to lose weight in a specific part of the body except to cut it off surgically. If you get the 5/5 response, however, the pounds will disappear from where you least want them—around your midsection. Your waistline will shrink inches, possibly overnight.

If addiction, appestat switch-off, or cravings are part of your problem, your weight should begin to melt away by the third day, as you break the addictions that have been causing you to overeat and discover which foods make you crave other foods or feel continually hungry. You may find out that the foods you thought were making you fat are not the real offenders.

Another factor that adds weight is sleeping, particularly the daily snooze that follows a hearty lunch. In many cases, the lethargy is an allergic reaction to what you've just eaten. Cut out the guilty food and the drowsiness will disappear.

The 5/5 AOD is less drastic than some regimes, but it calls for willpower and patience. You could have dramatic results within forty-eight hours if you're extremely food-allergic, or you could have no results at all. Fatigue and irritability may be a positive response, indicating that you're withdrawing from an addiction. If you feel wonderful, that's a good sign, too. It means that you're eliminating the foods that have been causing your symptoms.

Follow instructions—and no cheating, please. After the first two weeks, you should be feeling so good and losing so much weight that you won't want to cheat. If you find yourself craving a pizza or a candy bar, hold back. There's a 90 percent chance that it is some ingredient in that food—other than calories—that is making you fat.

When and if the craving strikes, take one gram (1,000 units) of Vitamin C every three hours until the desire subsides, or take alkali salts, or go for a walk in clean air. You can even do all three. Do anything but give in to your craving.

Be sure to weigh yourself daily and keep a diary of what you eat and drink and how you feel. Don't leave it to memory. And don't be surprised if you gain weight after eating a low-calorie food. You could be allergic to carrots, of all things, and a single bite might make you retain water.

The 5/5 AOD is divided into two parts: Preparation and Action. The first week of Preparation should ease you gently into Action.

PART 1: PREPARATION

Day 1: Eat anything you want except salt. Don't add it to your cooking or eat foods such as potato chips or bacon. Salt causes water retention, so if you don't stop eating it you won't know if it's salt or an allergic reaction that is making you bloated. Avoid salt for the duration of the diet.

Day 2: Same as Day 1.

Day 3: Eat anything you want (without salt) except for tap water. Drink pure bottled water or water that has been vigorously boiled for ten minutes; your system needs at least six glasses of fluid a day. Tap water may not have calories but it does contain compounds (chlorine, pesticides, salt) that can make you bloated. Drink pure water for the duration of the diet.

Day 4: Same as Day 3.

Day 5: Eat anything you want except sugar. Sugar is addictive, depletes the body of nutrients, and overworks the adrenal gland, which is necessary to resist allergy. It also feeds the growth of intestinal flora such as *Candida albicans,* but this is only a problem when you're allergic to the mold.

If you're in doubt about whether or not a product contains sugar, don't eat it. Anything ending in "ose" such as glucose, fructose, or dextrose is a sugar; corn syrup, corn sweeteners, molasses, and cane syrup should all be avoided.

The worst offenders are processed foods: Heinz Tomato Ketchup is 21 percent sugar; twelve ounces of Coca-Cola contain nine teaspoons of sugar; apple pie à la mode supplies eighteen teaspoons! Become a label watcher and avoid sugar for the duration of the diet. You may have two tablespoons of honey three times a week. Honey is the least chemically contaminated sweetener because bees exposed to pesticides rarely make it back to the hive.

Days 6 and 7: Same as Day 5.

PART 2: ACTION

This is the real beginning of the 5/5 AOD. Each week for the next five weeks you'll be eliminating one of the major food offenders: milk, wheat, eggs, corn, and yeast. Depending on the results, you'll either leave that food off your menus for the rest of the diet or reintroduce it at the end of the week.

Day 8: Continue the Preparation diet. *Eliminate cow's milk and cow's milk products.* This means you should avoid all obvious milk foods such as butter, cream, cheese, yogurt, most margarines, and buttermilk; any products that contain milk derivatives, such as lactose, casein, caseinate, sodium caseinate, lactoalbumin, lactoglobulin, curds, and whey; many baked goods, cakes, candies, chocolate, ice cream, sherbet, custards, donuts, cream sauces, cream soups, egg dishes, foods fried in butter, pancakes, waffles, mashed potatoes, macaroni, meatloaf, sausages, salami, bologna, frankfurters, and soufflés.

You can eat anything you want from Lists A and B of the Basic FSD plus wheat, eggs, corn, yeast, and their products, unless listed above. Drink six or more glasses of liquid a day, and be sure to replace any fluid that you would normally drink as milk.

Days 9–11: Same as Day 8.

Day 12: This is the fifth day of the Action part of your diet. Check your diary to see how much weight you have shed since Day 8. If you have lost five or more pounds in five days, the 5/5 response is a good indication that you are allergic to the specific food—in this case, milk—that you're eliminating.

Continue to avoid milk until you stop losing weight and reach a plateau. If that is your desired weight, you can end the diet. You know that milk makes you bloated and you should keep avoiding it. As long as you do, you should maintain your weight loss.

PART 1: PREPARATION

Day 1	Day 2	Day 3	Day 4	Day 5	Day 6	Day 7
Salt-free	Salt-free	Salt-free; no tap water	Salt-free; no tap water	Salt-free; no tap water; sugar-free	Salt-free; no tap water; sugar-free	Salt-free; no tap water; sugar-free

PART 2: ACTION (repeating days 1–7 and adding the following)

Day 8	Day 9	Day 10	Day 11	Day 12	Day 13	Day 14
Milk-free	Milk-free	Milk-free	Milk-free	Check for 5/5 reaction	Challenge test yourself	If no symptoms, reintroduce milk

REPEAT FOR A TOTAL OF FIVE WEEKS, REPLACING MILK-FREE WITH WHEAT-FREE, EGG-FREE, CORN-FREE, AND YEAST-FREE MENUS.

After two months, you can try reintroducing it into your meals. You may be able to tolerate a small amount at four-day intervals.

Day 13: If you did not get the 5/5 response, challenge yourself by drinking no more than a quarter of a glass of milk. Should you have a mild reaction—either immediate or delayed—take alkali salts, a gram of vitamin C, and possibly an antihistamine. A severe reaction, of course, requires prompt medical attention.

Day 14: If you did not gain weight overnight and have no other adverse symptoms, you may return milk to your diet.

Day 15: You're now starting a new week with a new food to eliminate. Continue the Preparation diet (no salt, sugar or tap water) but *cut out wheat and wheat products*. This means you should avoid all obvious wheat foods such as wheat flour, enriched, graham, or gluten flour, bran, hydrolized vegetable protein (HVP), and monosodium glutamate (MSG); any products that are thickened, such as gravy; all breads, cakes, cookies, crackers, pies, pastries, pretzels, and most breakfast cereals; pasta such as macaroni, spaghetti, and ravioli; ice cream cones and such beverages as Postum, Ovaltine, and malted milk; canned soups or any food containing noodles; sausage, hamburgers, meatloaf, and canned baked beans; alcoholic beverages such as beer, gin, or any drink containing grain neutral spirits.

You can eat anything you want from Lists A and B of the Basic FSD, plus milk (if you had no symptoms), eggs, corn, and yeast and their products, unless listed above.

Days 16–18: Same as Day 15.

Day 19: This is the fifth day of your wheat-elimination test. Have you lost five or more pounds in five days? If so, continue to avoid wheat until you reach a plateau. If that is your desired weight, you can end the diet and follow the instructions for Day 12.

Day 20: If you did not get the 5/5 response, try the challenge test: eat a cracker or any wheat product, and follow the instructions for Day 13.

Day 21: If you did not gain weight overnight and have no other adverse symptoms, you may return wheat to your diet.

Day 22: Repeat the same procedure as on Day 8, but *exclude eggs*. This means you should avoid all obvious egg products such as soufflés, custards, French toast, pastries, meringues, foods fried in batter, ice cream, mayonnaise, Hollandaise sauce, tartar sauce, marshmallows, root beer, prepared baking mixes, soups, sausage, meatloaf, foods containing albumin, vitellin, or ovovitellin, livetin, yolk, globulin, ovomucoid, ovomucin, and wine. You can eat anything from Lists A and B of the Basic FSD plus milk, wheat, corn, and yeast and their products, unless listed above.

Days 23–28: The same as Days 9–14, only substitute eggs for milk.

Day 29: Repeat procedure of Day 8, but *exclude corn.* This means you should avoid all obvious products such as corn flour, cornstarch, hominy grits, popcorn, corn flakes, corn syrups and sugars, mannitol and sorbitol (diet sweeteners), bacon, baking mixes and powders, white flour, breads and pastries, candies, carbonated beverages, cereals, some cheeses, instant coffee, cookies, eggnog, processed fish products, fried foods, French dressings, frostings, fruit drinks, graham crackers, gravy, chewing gum, ham, ice cream, jams, jellies, lemonade, margarines and shortenings, processed meats, monosodium glutamate (MSG), peanut butter, pickles, salad dressings, sandwich spreads, sauces, sherbets, soups and soup mixes, instant tea, tortillas, vinegar, and alcoholic beverages such as ale, beer, bourbon, gin, scotch, and most wines.

Additionally, corn is used as a binder in many tablets, liquids, and capsules; it is found in aspirin, breath sprays and drops, cough syrups, lozenges, ointments, suppositories, vitamins, laxatives, clothing starch, body and bath powder, and adhesives (don't lick envelopes, stamps, or stickers).

You can eat anything you want from Lists A and B of the Basic FSD plus milk, wheat, eggs, and yeast and their products, unless listed above.

Days 30–35: The same as Days 9–14, only substitute corn for milk.

Day 36: Repeat procedure of Day 8, but *exclude yeast.* This means you should avoid all baked goods containing yeast and all raised doughs such as breads and rolls; anything that contains mold, mushrooms, truffles, fungi, or fermented foods; all vinegar and products containing vinegar such as salad dressings, pickles, catsup, olives, many condiments, barbecue sauce, soy sauce, and chili sauce; tea; fermented beverages such as beer, wine, champagne, whiskey, brandy, tequila, beer, and ginger ale; any substances that contain alcohol, such as cough syrups; any kind of cheese, including cottage cheese, yogurt, buttermilk, and sour cream; all malt products; antibiotics and foods containing them, such as commercial beef, all dried fruits, nuts, and seeds and their products; spices, dried herbs, herb teas, and fruit juices unless home-squeezed.

You can eat anything you want from Lists A and B of the Basic FSD plus milk, wheat, eggs, and corn and their products, unless listed above.

Days 37–42: The same as Days 9–14, only substitute yeast for milk.

Day 43: You've been on this diet for over a month now, and you should be eating better, feeling better, and looking better. By cutting out salt, you will have automatically eliminated almost all processed foods from your menus; your new diet should be mostly fresh unprocessed foods with all their natural nutrients.

If you noticed no reaction to eliminating milk, wheat, corn, eggs, or yeast, you still may have food allergies. One indication is that you bloat more at certain times than others, or that you can gain two to five pounds overnight. You may be sensitive to foods not yet tried, such as pork, soy, coffee, chocolate, or citrus fruit.

A good way to find out is to make a list of all your favorite single foods. That would be apples, rather than apple pie; chicken, not chicken creamed in a patty shell. Mark the foods you would miss most if they were not in your diet. Then repeat the steps of Days 8–14 with your five favorite foods.

You should now have an excellent idea of what agrees or doesn't agree with you, and which foods make you gain weight. By eliminating your "fat" foods, and the edema, cravings, appestat switch-off, or addictive symptoms that go with them, you'll find you'll be able to take in many more calories than before without gaining an ounce.

Being allergic doesn't mean that you can't have delicious meals or that you'll enjoy eating any less. Once you wean your palate from salt and sugar, you'll find that your taste buds become exquisitely sensitive to natural flavorings, and that familiar foods take on new dimensions. One woman bit into a tomato while she was on the Basic FSD, and recalls, "It had the most delightful, sweet fruity taste. I don't think I had ever eaten a tomato before without salt or some kind of dressing."

Here are some ways to make life even sweeter.

COOKING HINTS

Sugar-Free

Honey comes in many different flavors: clover, orange blossom, rosemary, sage, and star thistle to name just a few. Each has its own character and flavor. Light-colored honeys tend to have more sweetness than taste and should be used when you don't want the honey flavor to come through. Dark-colored honeys tend to retain the taste of the flower or plant from which they were taken. The most popular mild flavors are star thistle, orange blossom, and sage.

Maple syrup and granulated maple sugar can be used instead of honey on your diet. Be sure to buy *pure* maple syrup and not maple "pancake" syrup, which contains corn sugar and artificial flavoring. Pour maple syrup over hot cereal or use as a glaze for meats and poultry. Granulated maple sugar works well for baking; substitute it in equal parts for white or brown sugar. It has a nutlike flavor.

Dried fruits and fruit juices also add sweetness. Try using dates minced in a blender or food processor. Make a purée of fresh bananas or soak dried fruit—apricots, pears, peaches, apples, raisins—in a small amount of water overnight and then purée. Frozen-juice concentrate is another good sweetener. Substitute fruit juice for liquids plus sugar when making desserts.

Milk-Free

Milk can be replaced in many recipes by a slightly smaller amount of water plus a teaspoonful of oil. Substitutes for butter include margarine (if it doesn't contain milk or artificial colors and flavors), or use any one of a number of cold pressed oils: olive, apricot kernel, avocado, walnut, sesame, safflower, sunflower. Each has its own subtle but distinct flavor. Kosher products such as margarine and bread are labeled "parve" when they don't contain milk.

Some other possible substitutes for cow's milk are:

Coconut milk. Considered a delicacy in many countries, it adds richness and sweetness to any recipe. To make it, purée a cup of fresh coconut meat with its own milk and extra water if needed for smoothness.

Goat's milk. Fresh goat's milk is often available in health-food stores, as are yogurt and over 200 varieties of goat cheeses, including goat's milk cheddar, Brie, Camembert, cream cheese, and any cheese such as *chèvre feuille* that contains the word *chèvre*—French for "goat." These have a strong flavor, so taste first before using goat products in a recipe.

Nut milks. These have long been used in European cuisine and by the American Indians. Almond and walnut milks are the most popular, but any nut can be used. They're excellent in sauces, puddings, and desserts. Prepare your own by soaking nuts in a small amount of water overnight. Blanching is optional. Purée in the blender, adding more liquid if necessary. Strain for purity or leave as is. Refrigerate.

Oat milk. Boil one cup of uncooked whole oat groats (not oatmeal) with five cups of water and a vanilla bean. Cover the pan and simmer one hour. Strain through a fine sieve or a thin cloth.

Seed milk. Soak seeds (such as sunflower) overnight in water or juice. Purée and strain.

Sheep's milk. Fresh sheep's milk is hard to find, but sheep's milk cheese is plentiful. Look for Roquefort (not all blue cheeses, only those specifically called Roquefort), feta, ricotta pecorino, or any cheese with the word *"pecorino"*—Italian for "sheep's milk cheese." Also available but not common is mozzarella made from buffalo milk.

Soy milk. This can be substituted cup for cup in any recipe calling for cow's milk and gives a similar taste and consistency. Buy it readymade or prepare it at home: gradually add one cup of soy flour to four cups of water in the blender. Strain, then heat drippings for twenty minutes in the top of a double boiler. Stir frequently. Cool and refrigerate.

Egg-Free

Eggs are important in recipes because they add volume and bind ingredients together. To replace an egg in baking, mix 1¼ tablespoons oil, 1¼ tablespoons water, and 1 teaspoon baking powder and add to recipe. If you need more than one egg, double, triple, or multiply amounts accordingly.

Wheat-Free

Wheat is used in baked goods because of its ability to rise and blend with other ingredients. Breads, cakes, and rolls made from other grains will have a denser texture.

Try substituting any of the following for one cup of wheat flour:

½ cup arrowroot
½ cup barley
¾ cup oats
1⅓ to 1½ cups ground rolled oats
¾ cup potato meal
⅝ cup potato starch
¾ to ⅞ cup rice flour
¾ to 1 cup rye flour
1 cup rye meal
¾ cup soybean flour

If you tolerate corn, replace one cup of wheat flour with:

1 cup corn flour
¾ cup corn meal (coarse)
1 scant cup corn meal (fine)
½ cup cornstarch

Combinations may give a more subtle flavor. These are also equivalent to one cup of wheat flour:

½ cup potato flour and ½ cup rye flour
⅓ cup potato flour and ⅔ cup rye flour
½ cup potato-starch flour and ½ cup soy flour
⅝ cup rice flour and ⅓ cup rye flour
1 cup soy flour and ¼ cup potato-starch flour

For thickening sauces and gravies, use the following foods. Mix with a little water before adding to gravy to help prevent lumps:

Arrowroot	1 tablespoon = 2½ tablespoons wheat flour
Barley flour	1 tablespoon = 1 tablespoon wheat flour
Cornstarch	½ tablespoon = 1 tablespoon wheat flour
Oatmeal	1 tablespoon = 1 tablespoon wheat flour
Potato Starch	½ tablespoon = 1 tablespoon wheat flour
Rice flour	½ tablespoon = 1 tablespoon wheat flour
Sago	½ tablespoon = 1 tablespoon wheat flour
Tapioca	½ tablespoon = 1 tablespoon wheat flour

Corn-Free

Corn-free diets are the easiest to cook for because corn products are not commonly found in recipes. Many baking powders contain cornstarch, though, so you may want to get a special corn-free brand at your natural-food store. Or substitute ½ teaspoon cream of tartar or ¼ teaspoon baking soda for 1 teaspoon baking powder.

Yeast-Free

Yeast is primarily used as a leavening agent in baked goods and has no equivalent replacement. Use recipes that call for baking soda or baking powder as leavening agents.

Grains such as barley, oats, and rye from the grass family or buckwheat from the buckwheat family are delicious when cooked in the same manner as rice and sweetened with dried fruits, honey, or maple syrup; sprinkled with chopped nuts; seasoned with herbs and spices; or mixed with vegetables. Many more ideas can be found in the cookbooks listed in the References section.

The hardest thing about eliminating any food is finding something to take its place. The best solution is to find new foods. Instead of becoming frustrated trying to bake a bread that tastes like your usual bread but doesn't contain wheat, explore other foods you've never tried before.

Continue to eat sensible meals and avoid your own particular fat foods. You'll soon find that you have a slimmer body, fewer allergic symptoms, and the happiness that goes with taking the first big step in helping yourself to health.

Chapter 5

HELP YOURSELF TO HEALTH

Now that you know your type, your symptoms, and many of the elements that provoke them, wouldn't it be nice if you could wave a wand and have all the allergy-causing substances in the world disappear? The trouble with that dream is that the earth and all its inhabitants would vanish, too. So why not make a simpler wish— that only the villains in your world disappear. To a great extent, that wish can come true. You can change your habits and material surroundings in ways that will raise your tolerance threshold, improve your resistance to illness and diseases, including allergy, and allow your immune system to function at full capacity.

Considering the immense quantities of pollens, petrochemicals, and various pollutants in the environment, it seems an overwhelming challenge. But the goal is to minimize exposure, not to lock yourself in a sterile cell with an oxygen tank.

CLEANING HOUSE

Start this program in a single room of your home or apartment, perhaps even the kitchen (if you don't have a gas stove), a bathroom, or a storage area. Get rid of molds, dust, and cleaning fumes, and then take a cot and sleep in there two or three nights to see if you feel better. If so, apply the same principles to your bedroom. That's the place you spend the most time, so it's the most important room in the house.

While you're playing detective, take note of the other rooms about you as well. Do you feel worse in the kitchen and better in the den? Wherever you feel bothered, look for a possible contaminant—something that isn't in the room where you feel good. Try to make a connection. If you can't, there are professional sleuths—"nontoxic-living consultants"—who make ecologic housecalls and bring their sharply trained noses right into your home to sniff out the culprits. You can get further information by writing to the Human Ecology Action League (HEAL) at 505 N. Lake Shore Drive, Suite 6505, Chicago, IL 60611. In the meantime, try as many of the following suggestions as you can, and to whatever extent possible.

The Type 1 Bedroom

For type 1 persons, the emphasis is on dust reduction.

1. Remove carpet or rugs; they are repositories of dust and molds. Waxed floors attract dust and keep some of it out of the air, but need to be cleaned more often with a vacuum or a wet mop. Use small throw rugs that are easy to wash.
2. Remove drapes and venetian blinds. Light, unlined washable curtains hold the least dust. Keep windows closed, especially during pollen season.
3. Check bedding. Avoid woolen blankets, feather pillows, down comforters, horsehair mattresses, and all fabrics derived from animals. Seal pillow and mattress in allergenproof covers to protect from dust and the highly allergenic dust mites that feed on the scales of skin you shed while you sleep. Wear a filter mask when you make your bed, let someone else make it, or leave it unmade.
4. Replace upholstered furniture with wood, metal, or canvas chairs. Do not use pillows, cushions, throws, dolls, or stuffed animals as decoration.
5. Remove all extraneous objects and furnishings. This includes bric-a-brac, scented products, plants or flowers, toys, pictures on walls, books, bookshelves, and mirrors unless they're flush. Bare is beautiful.
6. Keep all clothes in closets with the doors shut, or folded in drawers. Don't put clothes away dirty; they'll attract molds.

Let stored garments hang out in another room before wearing them.

7. Keep all pets, fish, and reptiles out of the bedroom, and out of the whole house if possible.

8. Do not allow smoking or smokers (whose hair, skin, and clothes carry smoke) into the bedroom.

9. Use an electric heater rather than gas, oil, or forced air. Keep the appliance clean, as heated or "fried" dust disintegrates into tiny particles that are easily inhaled. If your furnace uses forced air, close the ducts or seal them with aluminum foil and masking tape. Keep your bed away from the vent. Don't let the room temperature drop below 65 degrees, especially at night; air changes can trigger symptoms.

10. Get an air purifier. A small, inexpensive one does no good and may emit chemical contaminants. Look for an electrostatic precipitator or a high-efficiency particulate air filter (HEPA). Keep it on twenty-four hours a day with doors and windows closed. Try it on approval before buying it.

11. If it's possible to have someone else vacuum and dust your bedroom every day, by all means do so. If the responsibility is your own, wear a filter mask while cleaning, use a wet mop rather than a broom, and never empty a vacuum cleaner.

The Type 2 Bedroom

For Type 2 persons, the emphasis changes from dust reduction to chemical avoidance.

1. Remove carpet or rugs unless they're natural-fiber scatter rugs with no synthetic backing. Do not use wax, oil, or any polishing preparation on floor.

2. Replace drapes with rice-paper shades, metal blinds or screens, or untreated cotton curtains that have been washed in pure soap.

3. Check bedding. Eliminate all synthetic fibers such as polyester (Dacron) and foam rubber. Don't use an electric blanket, as the plastic wires tend to outgas when heated. Cotton, feather, and kapok pillows are fine for Type 2 persons, or use

a folded towel as a head rest. Your mattress should be encased in prewashed *barrier cloth* (tightly woven cotton; see "Where to Send for Products") and sewed together. Don't have any bedding professionally cleaned. Wash it at home in pure soap and water.

4. Replace upholstered or plastic furniture with chairs and tables made of wood, metal, or glass.

5. Remove all extraneous objects and furnishings. This includes cosmetic and other scented products, plants and flowers, anything made of plastic, books, bookshelves, newspapers, and magazines. If you're sensitive to newsprint, dry the item in the sunlight or carefully bake it—even a newspaper—for ten minutes in a 350-degree oven. Then read by an open window or an air filter, or use a special glass reading box (see "Where to Send for Products"). Appliances such as clocks, lamps, radios, telephones, television sets, and computers should be at least one year old.

6. Keep all clothes in closets with the doors shut, or folded in drawers. Don't keep any clothes in the bedroom that have been dry-cleaned, mothproofed, or washed in detergent. Drip-dry, permanent-press, or similarly finished clothes should not be in your wardrobe.

7. Do not allow smoking or smokers into the bedroom and, if possible, not anywhere in your house.

8. Do not permit friends or family members to enter your bedroom unless they are reasonably free of chemical odors, including deodorant, hair shampoo, and detergent-washed clothes.

9. If you have forced-air heating, gas and oils from the furnace can be toxic. Close the vent and seal with aluminum foil and aluminum duct tape. Use any one of three types of electric heater: radiant glass, a permanently sealed oil-filled portable radiator, or a hot-water baseboard unit. The last two are available in hardware and department stores. Any new portable heater should be turned on in another part of the house until the odor diminishes.

10. Open windows if you live in an unpolluted area. If you don't and there is no possibility you can move, get an activated-

carbon air filter to take chemicals out of the air. Keep it turned on by your bed, with doors and windows closed.

You may think some of these rules extreme; after all, dust supposedly doesn't bother Type 2 persons, and Type 1 persons don't react to scents. A Type 1 patient found out differently one morning when her family doctor made a housecall to treat her "virus" and commented on the strong smell of paint. The woman admitted that the fumes were all over the house, but assured him it was all right because she wasn't allergic to paint. At the same time, her throat was so hoarse she had to write notes.

The wise doctor explained that inhaling the strong odors was severely taxing her already-stressed immune system. He extracted a promise that all future paints would be latex acrylic, the least irritating, and that she would have the painter mix in one pound of baking soda per gallon of paint to help neutralize the fumes. He also suggested that she spend the next few nights at her parents' home, which she did. Her "virus" cleared up almost immediately.

Whatever your type, many everyday items are taxing your system, too, and increasing the number of stresses you carry. When the total load gets heavy enough, you may cross your tolerance threshold and suffer allergic symptoms.

Stop to ask yourself if you really need floral-scented hangers, peppermint mouthwash, and pine-spray air fresheners. Could you live happily ever after without fragrant facial tissues and perfumed toilet paper? The great American preoccupation with "smelling good" goes far beyond sanitation. Your drawers have to have floral sachets, your kitchen has to be "lemon-fresh," your bathroom has to reek of roses. The price tag for all these chemical scents is not in dollars alone.

Your body will be stronger, and the air you breathe and the world you live in will be healthier, if you reduce your and your family's consumption of odorous products. Not only should you try not to use them, you should seek, if possible, to remove them from your medicine cabinet, dressing tables, under sinks, and everywhere in the house.

High-fashion journals constantly brainwash their readers with such lines as "A home is not a home unless it's fragrant. Make life more sensual by smoothing a few drops of perfume onto your light bulbs. Tuck a perfumed-dampened cotton ball into your handbags, your writing paper, under your sheets." It's madness. Synthetic smells are getting in our hair and under our skin. Cologne-soaked blotters arrive in the mail with our bills, holiday presents appear in scented gift-wrap, paper dinner napkins smell like cherry pie, beautiful models spray us with God-knows-what as we stroll through department stores.

In August 1982 *OMNI* magazine reported that "olfactory manipulation has already begun" and described the commercial use of "spray-can-dispensed aromas designed to stimulate impulse purchases by customers. Aromas now available include a new car smell and the scents of fresh-baked bread and chocolate."

There's even something called *aroma therapy* in the wind, said to be derived from the Himalayan yogis' practice of using volatile plant essences to affect behavior, emotions, and disease. Dr. Robert I. Henkin, director of the Center for Molecular Nutrition and Sensory Disorders in Washington, D.C., reports that scientists are studying the body's olfactory mechanisms so that they can predict and affect human response to specific aromas. This could result in a "time-release canister" worn around the neck that emits pleasing odors at rush hour or other times of stress.

Also, "aromas could be specifically blended to cure insomnia or depression or to motivate people to work faster." In a mastery of understatement Henkin notes, "People might object to the fact that you are controlling their environment by pumping vapors into a room through the air-conditioning duct."

Indoor pollution is one of the major health issues of the 1980s, according to California's former consumer affairs director, Richard Spohn. In 1982 his department issued a 600-page report listing some of the prime causes: asbestos in insulation; formaldehyde in carpeting and walls; radon, a radioactive gas used in energy-efficient building materials; hundreds of thousands of consumer products ranging from aerosol sprays to shoe polish; tobacco smoke. The report wisely suggested a requirement for cigarettes to be self-extinguishing.

It will and should come. The deleterious effects of cigarette smoke are cumulative. It has taken fifty years to uncover the dramatic increase of diseases caused by this habit, but there is no longer any room for doubt. Nonsmokers, particularly allergic ones who have been forced by economic pressures to be exposed to cigarette smoke in their work environment, are suffering more severe allergies, arthritis, and other debilitating or life-threatening diseases due primarily to prolonged inhalation of this potent toxin.

Just as people have become supersensitive to tobacco smoke in the last few decades, so will they soon become intolerant of synthetic scents. Guests will begin to request "nonperfumed" dinner partners and fragrance-free sections in restaurants; hostesses will set out charming needlepoint pillows that say, "In This House No One Makes Scents"; politicians will race to be the first to write antiodor laws; prospective lovers will ask each other, "Do you spray?"

No matter what you see on television, personal hygiene needn't come in fancy packages or leave you smelling like crushed strawberries, and doesn't have to be expensive to be good. Phyllis Diller had the right perspective when she said, "Cosmetics can do wonders for a woman. Look what they did for Elizabeth Arden, Merle Norman, and Estée Lauder."

The Food and Drug Administration requires complete listings of ingredients on domestic cosmetics, but how many people know what propylene glycol, isotearyl neopentanoate, or titanium dioxide are? Labels mean almost nothing to the average consumer, so you must fall back on a single rule: smell the product. The stronger the odor, the less should be your inclination to buy it.

Odors from synthetic chemicals, in small amounts, are harmless for most people. But for Type 2 persons, and occasionally for Type 1 persons as well, these fumes have the capacity to damage the immune system, cause it to malfunction, and result in an intolerance to the chemical products. The substances that bother susceptible people are the ones they use most frequently: makeup, deodorant, soap, cologne, and aftershave.

Once you become sensitized to a substance, your immune system will be less tolerant of other chemical substances, and you may experience more symptoms. On the other hand, you may be able to use a single deodorant or shampoo all your life without becoming sensitized.

A product does not have to smell to be effective. Baking soda is the best dentifrice you can use to clean teeth, as well as an all-purpose deodorant, an excellent kitchen and bathroom cleanser, an effective mouthwash, and a spot remover for carpets. It has no odor.

Most cosmetics are available unscented, or can be replaced with a natural (nonsynthetic) product. You can easily learn to shampoo your hair with a blend of two eggs and two tablespoons of vodka; or to cleanse your skin with fresh yogurt; or to rub on sesame oil as a sunscreen.

The same is true of home maintenance. Lemon juice will shine brass, copper, and aluminum; white vinegar will clean windows, tubs, and showers; vegetable oils will polish shoes and furniture. All odors are natural and all products are cheaper, safer, and better for your health than their synthetic counterparts. See "Where to Send for Products" for sources of other safe supplies.

Clothing occasionally causes problems for allergic people. Some Type 1 persons can't tolerate anything made of animal hair or feathers, or woven from grasses. The same "natural fibers"— cotton, linen, silk, and wool—are highly desirable for Type 2s, as long as the materials don't have chemical finishes.

A finish is the treating of a fabric to make it more salable. It affects either the looks or the performance. Scotch-Guard, for instance, is a finish that protects from soiling; other finishes repel water, retard flames, and maintain permanent press. These treatments make materials very practical to consumers, but they also emit toxic vapors that can irritate the chemically sensitive. In many cases, the finishes can be removed by laundering or by overnight soaking in baking soda or vinegar.

Whether you're a Type 1, a Type 2, or a combination of both, you will benefit from living in a home that's well ventilated and free of contaminants. And if this is true of the home environment, think how essential it is in the typical modern office.

ALLERGENS AT WORK

How do you tell your boss that you'd love to make copies of his memo but every time you go near the copy machine you get depressed? Your employer would either laugh, scowl, or dispatch you to the company shrink.

Gradually, that situation is changing. Much has been written about the hazards of working in the modern office, the toxic properties of seemingly innocent vapors, and the increase of illnesses associated with energy-sealed buildings that don't allow these gases to escape. Mental symptoms such as confusion and depression are becoming too common to ignore, and the enlightened boss, faced with an employee's plea for understanding, is much more likely to listen and be sympathetic than he was in the past.

Your employer is now required by law to ensure that you have healthful working conditions, that you're trained to do your job safely, and that you're given whatever protective gear you need. Everyone who handles any kind of machine or equipment, from the simplest manual typewriter to the most sophisticated computer, is a potential work-disability target. Whether or not you become one depends on:

How allergic you are, particularly to chemicals or dust

Degree and duration of exposure

Your age, sex, and heredity

Whether you smoke

Your diet and other habits

Your home environment

Your general physical condition

Two of the most common office offenders are the ubiquitous copy machine and the VDT, or video display terminal. VDTs are small desk computers widely used by all kinds of businesses, newspapers, hospitals, government bureaus, and schools.

In March 1982 William E. Murray of the National Institute for Occupational Safety and Health pointed out the lack of scientific knowledge about possible ill effects of ultraviolet, radio frequency, and X-radiation from VDTs, and admitted the need for research despite "theoretical reasons" for believing that the human body does not absorb low-frequency radiation.

VDTs have been known to cause vision deterioration, headaches, irritation, back pains, dizziness, and excessive fatigue in up to 75 percent of the estimated 15 million Americans who use them on a daily basis. Recent studies have uncovered one reason why. The face of the screen carries a charge of positive ions that draws negative ions from the surrounding area. Approximately eighteen inches of space between the screen and the operator's face are relatively devoid of air ions. This changes the membrane charge of the nasal mucosa cells and starts a reaction that affects the person's whole body.

To avoid this, the operator should use a detached keyboard and sit at least twenty inches from the monitor, open the window, or use a fan to blow fresh air across the screen. Specially treated film on the VDT face will also alleviate the problem.

Type 2 persons may react to the outgassing of the heated plastic components, particularly in a modern energy-sealed office. Continued exposure to low-energy radiation can damage the immune system and exacerbate allergic symptoms in both types.

Thus low radiation exposure, air devoid of ions, vision problems, and the constrained postures of VDT workers combined with chemical fumes in the workplace, stagnant air, the monotony of repetitive tasks, and normal business stresses do not add up to the kind of environment in which a person can build up his immune system to fight allergies.

Yet the Type 1 or Type 2 person who can use the VDT in a ventilated and properly lit room, who has adequate back support, who does reasonably challenging work, and does not have to sit there all day may find that, if he eats wisely and spends the rest of his time in a nontoxic environment, he may be perfectly healthy.

The photocopier presents a different challenge to the allergic person because of inks and solvents that permeate the surrounding air. Combine these fumes with cigarette smoke in a building with hermetically sealed windows that can't be opened, and you have an atmosphere that can irritate both Type 1 and Type 2 persons.

You can best prevent this situation by trying to ensure that copy machines are in well-ventilated areas or near windows that can be opened. Copiers and all machines that emit chemical fumes should be rigged so that their gases flow into the building's exhaust system. Empty toner bottles and other copy machine waste products should be disposed of separately rather than in the office trash basket. If you have to touch or breathe any photocopying chemicals, you may want to wear gloves or a mask. Even the paper is often coated with materials that can cause skin or lung reactions.

Occupational dermatitis, according to the National Safety Council, costs Americans more than $100 million annually in lost work hours and medical bills. Skin rashes can erupt in response to almost every type of supply or equipment from typewriter ink to plastic desk tops.

Cigarette smoking accounts for an estimated $13 billion in health-care expenses, according to the California Nonsmokers' Rights Foundation, and not a small part of that figure goes for health problems developed by nonsmokers. The organization warns that children of smoking parents have more allergic manifestations than children of nonsmoking parents. Type 1 respiratory symptoms are unquestionably aggravated by smoke, and Type 2 cerebral symptoms are often triggered by one or a combination of the 4,600 chemicals contained in tobacco fumes. Secondhand smoke can make allergic persons more sensitive to other substances or push a nonreacting person over his tolerance threshold. The American Medical Association estimates that 34 million Americans are sensitive to tobacco smoke. Twice that figure would probably be more accurate.

Another office hazard is that some building owners try to save money and fuel by running ventilation systems at half-power, or only for certain hours of the day. When the flow slows down, the air collects dust from dirt and chemicals, and workers end up inhaling these toxic particles.

Severely allergic persons may have no choice but to change workplaces or even occupations. There is no healthy future for a Type 1 person working in a carpenter shop full of sawdust, in a pet store abounding in animal dander, or in a flower nursery heavy with pollens. A Type 2 garage mechanic, house painter, or beautician would fare equally poorly breathing the fumes of his profession. The ideal work for any allergic person is either self-employment (writer, tailor, composer, private tutor, shopowner, etc.), as long as *you* control the materials and the environment, or a job where your employer allows you to have an office at home.

If neither alternative is possible, try to pick a suitable location. Type 1 persons might breathe more easily in a new building full of plastics and synthetics as long as it's relatively dust-free, is sealed against outside air containing pollens, and has sufficient indoor ventilation. Air conditioning could help to keep temperatures warm and constant, which would be nice for Type 1 persons, even though the system's components are chemically cleaned to stop mold growth. The air of a large metropolitan city, polluted as it is, would probably be less irritating to a Type 1 than the dusty, pollen-heavy air in the country.

Type 2 persons should seek older buildings with steam or electric heat, wood or hard linoleum floors, and windows that open. Preferably, such a building should be situated far from congested urban areas, not only because of the poor air available for office ventilation but also because of all the fumes involved in traveling to and from work. In downtown areas, offices on higher floors are preferred since they receive less traffic exhaust through open windows.

Type 2 persons (and any Type 1 who so desires) can minimize chemical exposure in the office by following these suggestions:

1. Don't smoke, and ask your fellow employees not to smoke around you. If they refuse, talk to your employer. You have a legal right to a healthful working environment.

2. Ask your fellow workers not to wear strong scents or hairspray. This is a touchy request, but if you ask gently and take time to explain your situation (with a smile and perhaps a gift of unscented soap or shampoo), you may get cooperation.

3. Try to avoid proximity of copiers, mimeographs, or other machines that use solvents. Get a friend to operate them for you when necessary.

4. If you must operate a machine that requires inks or solvents, keep an air purifier in the office.

5. Try to keep office furniture free of foam rubber, plastic, and synthetic upholstery. Wood or metal are best.

6. Correction tape is better than correction fluid, glue sticks are preferable to rubber cement, and carbon paper makes less toxic copies than NCR (No Carbon Required) paper or machines.

7. Give freshly printed or duplicated pages a chance to dry before handling or reading them.

8. Request that pesticides and strong cleaning solvents not be used in your area. If this is impossible, consider doing your own cleaning with acceptable products.
9. Use odorless pens and markers, staples and metal paper clips instead of tape or glue, and wood or metal (not plastic) desk accessories.
10. Insist that all construction and remodeling be done when no office workers are around. Fumes from such labors must be dissipated before you and your co-workers inhabit the air space.

Some observers say that the popular "Thank God It's Friday" euphoria has more to do with escaping office pollutants than with relief from psychological stress. "Getting away for the weekend" makes many people feel energetic, alive, and free of symptoms, and, if so, your feelings may be more physical than mental, especially if you go home to a clean atmosphere. When you go elsewhere for a weekend or for a longer vacation, there are other factors you'll want to think about.

TIPS FOR TRAVEL

The definition of travel, as used here, includes every thing from driving to the country for the day to circling the globe. Each time you leave your front door, you encounter an environment full of challenges. The substances you touch, eat, smell, and breathe outside the home all hold potential allergens. They may be better than what you live with indoors, or they may cause new problems.

Wherever you go, try to choose a destination as free of your particular allergens as possible. Seashores and mountains seems to be the most beneficial vacation spots for both Type 1 and Type 2 persons; the air is crisp, clear, and holds few industrial pollutants or pollens.

Keep in mind that all allergic people are particularly susceptible to damage from parasites or viral infection. These ailments can be cured, but they intensify allergies and can leave you with years of problems. A patient once shrugged: "I might as well eat the native food in Nepal. If I get anything, I'll just take antibiotics." He was informed that he could rid himself of the organism, but the damage it would do to his immune system could last a lifetime.

The best way to avoid germs is to keep yourself as clean as possible and free of excess hair. Men who grow beards, especially in the tropics, offer attractive housing to fungi and parasites. Crowds are good places to pick up infections, and hence are good places to avoid for many reasons. Allergic persons do not benefit from inhaling perfume, tobacco, cosmetic, deodorant, and sunscreen scents, animal dander, food smells, or any of the other odors that waft through gatherings of people.

When and where to eat can be a problem for both Type 1 and Type 2 persons, especially if all your meals are in restaurants. Ask for a nonsmoking section as far as possible from the kitchen's fumes and gases. You needn't be afraid to request that the chef prepare your chicken, fish, or salad with only the ingredients you specify. Better restaurants, where most foods are cooked fresh and à la carte, are more likely to respect your wishes.

If you've ever had severe asthma, intense reactions to drugs or insect stings, or strong responses to foods or chemicals, you will want to carry a wallet card and wear a dogtag or wrist band with your medical information. This will protect you from the wrong kind of treatment in an emergency. Medic Alert (P.O. Box 1009, Turlock, CA 95380) is a nonprofit foundation that supplies these items for a $15 fee. Or you can send $16.50 to Micro-Design Systems (P.O. Box 11, 15 Broad Street, Boston, MA 02110) for a device called Mediscope. It reproduces your medical history on microfilm and encases it in a neck pendant. You hold the piece up to a light and look through the magnifying lens at the top.

Now let's discuss specific travel situations.

When Type 1 Persons Travel

The outdoor well-being of a Type 1 person generally has to do with temperature changes, whether or not the plants are blooming, how much dampness, dryness, and dust are in the air, and the force of the wind. Leaving town during hay fever season is a good idea if you know where you're going. Your destination should be a place where your particular allergens do not thrive, and at a time when few plants are pollinating. You should also have the option to leave if you're bothered. Some people seek the sun and warmth of the desert only to find that the hot, dry air hardens mucous membranes and makes their respiratory symptoms worse.

Transportation should be a prime consideration. Will you go by boat, plane, train, car, or bus? If by water, remember that lakes and rivers tend to gather algae and pollens on their surfaces and are often bordered by grasses. Oceans have no pollens and are ideal for Type 1 persons. If you can afford any deep-water cruise in a warm climate, be it on a freighter or the *Royal Viking Star*, take it, and spend as much time as possible breathing on deck. One patient's two-week voyage was near-miraculous. The ocean air did what no antihistamine had ever been able to do: it cleared her stuffy sinuses in three days.

An antihistamine/decongestant can be most effective on an airplane if you take it at least half an hour before you board. It will keep your nasal passages clear and reasonably unaffected by pressure changes. Chewing sugarless gum at takeoff and landing helps, too. And since planes are often overly air conditioned, you may need warm clothing.

New trains and buses offer more conveniences than old ones, and are freer of dust and molds. Air conditioning in vehicles sometimes spreads pollutants, especially mold spores, and the chilled draft can aggravate your respiratory passages. But air conditioning can work for you, too. If you have access to the thermostat, turn it up and keep your cabin or compartment at a warm, even temperature.

Type 1 persons travel best in well-maintained automobiles that are not full of pet hairs, debris, or tobacco smoke. Some national agencies, such as Thrifty Rent-A-Car, now offer choices of "smoking" or "nonsmoking" cars, and find that the majority of their customers prefer cars driven by nonsmokers. Choose your route carefully, aiming for coast or mountain highways rather than inland roads through farm country.

Where you stay can be a problem if not planned. Any modern hotel is preferable to a farm, ranch, or country-style resort. A small "family-type" pension or bed-and-breakfast inn may sound quaint and charming, but is liable to have chickens or pets, plants and flowers, ruffled curtains, bric-a-brac, overstuffed chairs, and other dust catchers. A place that's "cozy" is a place to avoid.

In fact, most Type 1 persons who have been houseguests feel they'd rather stay in hotels. The extra dollars are worth the convenience of having a situation you can control. You can't ask a hostess to turn up the heat if everyone else is comfortable. You can't very well complain about the pine wood in the fireplace, your freshly painted room, or the vase of roses so thoughtfully placed by your bed. But those lovely personal touches can make you miserable.

Generally speaking, a traveling Type 1 fares better on land and sea than in the air, in modern hotels rather than in private homes, and in cities and countries that are more civilized and sophisticated than they are primitive. Leave the dusty ruins and moldy subterranean caves for the archeologists.

When Type 2 Persons Travel

The picture completely reverses itself for Type 2 persons, whose first consideration must be an area free of urban and industrial pollutants. Your well-being doesn't have much to do with the time of year, except that you don't belong anywhere in "tourist season," where drip-dry and perma-press fabrics abound and tend to outgas in warm weather. Your destination should be a place with a cool or moderate climate, preferably in the country, in the mountains, or by a large body of water. Bustling cities are not recommended.

Getting where you're going may be something of a challenge. Luxury cruise liners would be fine if you could sleep in the fresh air on deck. But the cabins of newer ships are mainly made of synthetics, and the people who clean them carry enough spray bottles to sanitize an army. Disinfectants reek through the corridors and blow through the air-conditioning system so that the cleanliness of the ship is often in direct proportion to the pollution of the indoor air. A passenger once asked a stewardess why she had to spray the furniture in order to dust it. She replied that that was what they were told to do because it was "more thorough." Older ships, freighters, and less luxurious vessels would probably have fewer chemical problems.

The major airlines are usually gracious when alerted to a passenger's special needs. If you're bothered by airport fumes, you can call ahead, arrange to check in at the curb, and board the plane early. Your clinical ecologist can provide (or tell you where to get) a small charcoal-filtered breather that will help you handle the exhaust gases around the airport.

If you have to layover in an airport and the air is particularly heavy with gas or smoke fumes, look for the infirmary or first-aid station, or tell the airline representative you are having trouble breathing and cannot stay there. Airlines often have private waiting areas for special passengers.

Trains and buses mean unavoidable exposure to a variety of airborne irritants, starting with very potent diesel fumes. Try to sit with the windows closed in the least-polluted air—towards the rear of trains and in the front of buses. Trains usually have nonsmoking sections but buses offer no such protection.

One Type 2 patient just back from a trip reports, "I spent a day on Amtrak and the train was terrific because there were no fumes and the whole car was nonsmoking. I also liked the New York subway. No fumes there, either, even underground, and the trains had plastic seats but no cushions, synthetic fibers, or rugs like the San Francisco BART trains do. It was much better than sitting in a taxi in traffic. I think trains are the best transportation for people with chemical allergies. They're less crowded, too."

No public transportation, alas, can shield you from the clothing, cosmetic, and food scents of the other passengers. You may have more control in an automobile, particularly one that's several years old and doesn't smell of vinyl or newly treated leather.

Ideally, your car should be lightweight, which means it consumes less gas, and should not have been used by heavy smokers. Type 2 persons feel best sitting in the front seat, away from the exhaust, and near an open window if the air is clear. Sunroofs also provide ventilation suitably distant from exhaust fumes. Heavy vehicles give off the most gases, so you should avoid trailing mobile homes, trucks, and buses. Keep a good distance between you and the other car ahead, and, if possible, travel at night when traffic is sparse.

Choosing a route is as important as the right vehicle. Look for less-traveled secondary highways far from the flow of traffic, and plan your drive so that you don't pass through factory areas. If possible, try to avoid construction zones, new roads with fresh tar, land that has recently been sprayed with pesticide, and burning fields that are releasing vapors. Exposure to any of these allergens could result in immediate cerebral symptoms that might impair memory and judgment, cause overpowering fatigue, and—if you're driving—put you to sleep at the wheel. A charcoal air filter that plugs into the lighter socket might be a worthwhile investment to protect against this possibility.

Your hotel should be exactly what the Type 1 doesn't want: a small family-type dwelling, a bed-and-breakfast inn, a country ranch. If the owners grow their own fruits and vegetables, beware of pesticides and fertilizers. Expensive older hotels should be no problem, as they're built with wood, marble, and concrete rather than synthetics—and their windows open. Get as high a room as you can for the cleanest air, and stay far away from the swimming pool. When you call for reservations, be sure to ask if the hotel has recently been renovated. If so, don't stay there.

Again, a private home is not recommended unless you know the owner well, and he or she understands your problem. It's not easy to ask your hostess to remove the synthetic carpets, turn off her natural gas furnace, or drain the pool of chlorinated water.

Type 2 persons probably fare best traveling by land or sea in older vehicles, staying in places considered quaint, countrified, or historical landmarks, and visiting rural areas, seaside communities, mountain resorts, or islands of anthropological and cultural interest.

Many allergic people find that vacationing at the right time and in the right places brings not only relief of symptoms but also insight into some of the culprits they left behind. Others find that traveling aggravates their symptoms and makes them wonder if their allergies may be too complicated to handle alone. If so, they have a logical recourse.

CHOOSING A DOCTOR

There comes a time in the life of every allergic person when you must decide whether your symptoms are severe enough to require the services of a specialist or whether you should "learn to live with them." Only you can make this decision. The mildly allergic person, particularly a Type 1, can often exist happily and in good health simply by avoiding lobsters and German shepherds. If you know what your allergies are, and the situations or conditions that provoke them, you may get along fine with a few antihistamines and a box of tissues.

If your symptoms are more severe or perplexing and have not been sufficiently helped by diet and environmental changes, take heart. There's no reason to consign yourself to a life of illness and discomfort. Medical care is at the other end of your telephone. Your chances of getting well in the hands of a physician you mistrust or dislike, however, or who is too busy or uninterested to develop a rapport, are negligible. For this reason, your choice of a doctor must be a careful one. You wouldn't pick a brain surgeon from the Yellow Pages, and neither should you trust your allergic well-being to a toss of the dice.

With allergy, more than almost any other illness, you, the patient, are responsible for how fast and how well you progress. The question, then, is how to choose a doctor who will be open-minded, knowledgeable, and able to create a mood of concern and optimism. He must be someone who treats you as a person, not as a Type 1 or a Type 2, and not merely as a list of symptoms or a case history. He must give you the feeling that at the moment he is attending you, you and your health are all that matter. Most of all, he must be able to motivate you to make changes in your diet and lifestyle.

The allergist's role is to guide you back to health by achieving three goals: accurate diagnosis, proper treatment, and the mobilization of your own healing resources. If he fails at any one of these functions, he fails altogether. Self-healing may be the most important factor, since your recovery depends on your will to restore your immune system to normal efficiency and to take the necessary steps outside the doctor's office to get well.

Your first act should be to consult your family doctor. He knows you and your symptoms better than anyone, and belongs to an active medical network. He knows which of his patients have been helped by which specialists and which have not. He's aware of his colleagues' reputations, and even though personal likes and dislikes can't be discounted, he's got your welfare at heart.

So ask him for a recommendation. After reading the previous chapters, you're well aware that there are two kinds of allergists—

154 The Type 1/Type 2 Allergy Relief Program

those who observe traditional methods and those who practice clinical ecology.

How Physicians Differ

Basically speaking, the two doctors are not that dissimilar. Both agree that:

Avoidance is the best treatment for all allergies.

Scratch tests are generally reliable for inhalants and unreliable for foods.

Blood tests, as structured today, are mainly unreliable but can be useful when nothing else is available.

Immunotherapy—building up the immune system with antigens so that the body's own defenses can withstand allergens—is the best treatment after avoidance.

Allergies can be helped by medical treatment, and, in many cases, will completely disappear.

But the doctors also have their disagreements. Conventionalists believe in using drugs and medication as an adjunct to immunotherapy. Clinical ecologists believe medication should be a last resort.

Conventionalists do not believe that the results of sublingual therapy have been proven or documented, or that neutralization—that is, turning off an acute reaction with a lower dose of the same antigen that caused it—is a scientific fact. Most of them deny the existence of Type 2 chemical allergies and do not believe that chemicals can produce such mental disorders as schizophrenia.

Traditional practitioners feel that untreated allergies can lead to severe lung problems such as chronic bronchitis or emphysema, whereas clinical ecologists see allergies as forerunners of such serious immune system disorders as rheumatoid arthritis, multiple sclerosis, and cancer.

Once you know how the two allergists think you can better choose your specialist. As stated before, there is no difference in basic immunological philosophy: both use antigen therapy to build up T cells. The difference is in testing and treating. The conventional practitioner will scratch forty to ninety antigens on your back, make a diagnosis, and start you right away on injections. The clinical ecologist will spend several days finding the exact neutralizing dose for each substance to which you react.

Type 1 patients have been and continue to be successfully treated by conventional allergists, and if your problems are mainly localized, seasonal, or respiratory, you may want the traditional approach. Conventional allergists rarely treat chemical allergies or even acknowledge that they are more than occasional irritants to the skin and respiratory system.

Be warned that your family doctor may not be familiar with the principles of clinical ecology and may be reluctant to recommend this alternative. His caution is understandable, since the field is just now becoming "legitimized" as scientists identify more and more of the basic mechanisms that cause chemical allergies. But your doctor should be open-minded and willing to make inquiries.

If he becomes impatient or angry, is closed to new ideas, or offers to send you to a psychiatrist, find a more compassionate family doctor. There is no question that a significant number of patients who suffer mental and behavioral symptoms would benefit from astute psychiatric treatment, but many of these patients would benefit even more from proper allergy treatment.

The names of reputable clinical ecologists in your area may be obtained by writing to the Society for Clinical Ecology (SCE) at 2005 Franklin Street, Suite 490, Denver, CO 80205.

Costs

Both types of allergist charge $80 or more for an initial consultation and $200 or more for the first round of testing, which doesn't include laboratory tests or X-rays. Most procedures are covered by medical insurance.

Desensitizing injections from a traditionalist will cost about $15 a week, plus another $200 or so for a year's supply of antigens. You'll need more antigen solution for the weekly, daily, or several-times-a-day sublingual applications that the clinical ecologist prescribes, but you'll save the price of office visits and injections. Whichever allergist you choose, you can expect to pay

$1,000, more or less, for the first year of treatment, and perhaps half as much the second year.

Be prepared, too, to have the clinical ecologist urge radical changes in your lifestyle. The traditionalist may tell you to vacuum your bedroom rug more often and take antihistamines; the clinical ecologist will say that the rug has to go, particularly if it's synthetic and you're a Type 2. Such major adjustments are costly but, for most people, result in fewer symptoms and fewer long-range medical expenses.

Clinical ecology treatment is faster and should make you feel better within two to four weeks. Most practitioners believe that in one or two years you may not need further medical care. Traditional allergists generally advocate a maintenance program of monthly (or so) hyposensitization injections throughout your lifetime.

What to Expect at the Office

You may be surprised the first time you enter a clinical ecologist's office. The waiting room will probably have wooden or canvas-backed chairs, no cushions, no carpet, steam heating from a radiator, an air filter, and a large NO SMOKING sign. If the office has a copier and a computer-printer, they are located out of the patients' sight and smell in a well-ventilated corner or a separate room. The magazines are too old to emit newsprint fumes, the receptionist's desk is devoid of colored marking pens, glues, or plastic containers. A cooler containing spring water is available to anyone who is thirsty and, somewhere within reach, there's a green metal tank in case pure oxygen is needed.

All staff personnel wear cotton, silk, or wool clothing. They don't use scents, nail polish, or hairspray. Very often these people have been drawn to the field because of their own allergies.

Whether you're a Type 1 or Type 2, the procedure is the same: the clinical ecologist will first take a complete and extremely detailed history, concentrating on both past and present symptoms. Be prepared by asking parents or relatives what you were like as an infant. Did you cry a lot? Did you have any unusual physical or mental problems? Were you a colicky baby? How did you tolerate childhood diseases and vaccinations? What were your eating habits as a child?

The doctor may even go back to your mother's pregnancy, since drugs taken and illnesses suffered at that time often alter the fetus' immune system and can show up as disease thirty or forty years later. He will ask about your weight pattern, your reactions to weather and seasonal changes, your mental state and moods. If you've had a general anesthetic, he'll say, "Do you have positive, negative, or neutral feelings about going under again?" Your answer tells him if you reacted adversely to the anesthetic, even as long as twenty years ago.

You'll be queried about every illness from the most minor viral infection to emergency surgery, and the doctor will want to know your feelings about your treatment, and if you feel you've completely recovered. He may pose such seemingly trivial questions as: Do you have a garden? Do you keep pets? Where do you work? What tools or instruments do you use? Do the windows in your office or building open? Do you travel by car or bus? Do you bring your lunch or eat in the cafeteria? Are there any foods that you can't live without, such as chocolate, Coca-Cola, whole-wheat bread, or eggs?

In short, he seeks answers from you rather than from his orthodox medical training, which taught a great deal about medication and surgery but very little about the human body's subtle interactions with the environment.

Questions You Should Ask

Prepare to interrogate your allergist, be he conventionalist or clinical ecologist. Don't hesitate to ask any of these questions that apply:

What are your fees? Do you require payment at the time of treatment? Will my bill be itemized?

What did you find out from the physical examination? (Unless it's an emergency, accept no medication or treatment if the doctor has not done a complete physical.)

What kind of lab tests have you ordered and what do you hope to learn from them?

Are X-rays absolutely necessary? Why? (Doctors now suggest you keep records of all X-rays, including dental, and when and where taken. Then you will have some idea of how much radiation you've had.)

How will you test me and for what substances? (Be sure he includes all the things you suspect.)

How will you treat me? What is immunotherapy? Does it work for everyone? (Statistics show that antigen therapy by drops or injection successfully desensitizes 75 percent of the patients who try it.)

Why is this drug indicated for me? How does it work in the body? Does it have any side effects? Is there an alternative to drug therapy?

If not, what is the minimum dosage I can take? Does it react with other foods, medicines, or alcohol? How soon can I expect results? How long should I continue taking it? If I feel better, may I stop the drug? Can I save money by ordering it in generic form?

You have a right to know what's going on in your body, and a good doctor will respect your questions and answer them seriously. If you feel he has rushed you, is careless about returning phone calls, or can't be bothered with your queries, it's up to you to tell him so. You're paying well for his services and you should be getting them.

Never feel it's disrespectful to challenge your doctor's judgment about a procedure. He welcomes dialogue with his patients and prefers that you be fully aware of the treatment course. Sometimes, fortunately rarely, even the best doctor can make a mistake, and an astute patient will catch the error before it causes problems. If you feel your questions are resented, find another doctor.

Both types of allergist may have so many patients that they treat you like a car on a production line. They see you once, on the first visit, and then turn you over to a technician for a battery of routine tests. The technician diagnoses your allergies, arranges treatment, supplies a few printed sheets of instructions, and sends you out to face the world. You continue to see the technician, not the doctor, until you specifically complain or ask for another appointment. If you're not helped, the doctor may even be irritated or blame you for not following instructions. In most cases, he'll return you to the technician and run you through the assembly line again.

A good allergist may have a staff of technicians, but he supervises every stage of your progress and lets you know he's available *at all times* if you have questions or problems.

Dr. Marvin Belsky, author of *How to Choose and Use Your Doctor*, observes: "The informed patient takes a stake in his treatment. He feels confident about monitoring his well-being. He expresses his doubts to his doctor, and he doesn't act until he has been convinced beyond a reasonable doubt that the course he's electing is the right one. He does all this together with his doctor."

Today's patients are better educated than they've ever been, more aware of their rights, more desirous of information, and more familiar with treatment techniques. They know not to except or demand instant relief, they realize that many allergies can be helped but not cured, and they no longer feel that they have to leave a doctor's office with pills or prescriptions.

This is quite a departure from the longtime assumption that a patient doesn't feel "treated" unless he leaves a doctor's office with pills or medication. Scientists have long known that healing processes are closely involved with the brain. They are just beginning to realize what a potent ally the mind can be in the struggle against allergies. And there are many old and new ways to harness these brain energies.

Chapter 6

ALTERNATIVE TREATMENTS

Allergies respond not only to avoidance, immunotherapy, and medication but to a variety of currently popular mind and body disciplines. Creative patients, some who have tried medical treatment and some who haven't, are turning to new techniques such as biofeedback and visualization, as well as to the ancient arts of acupuncture and hypnosis. Long scorned as fads or trends of the moment, many of these treatments are earning respect and respectability, even from conservative members of the medical profession.

One advantage of these methods is that they apply to both types of allergy, and to mild cases as well as to severe ones. Also, they have no direct side effects, are easily available, are usually inexpensive, and some can even be self-taught. They often work when conventional treatment has failed, or as an adjunct to medical care to heighten and enhance its effects.

MIND TECHNIQUES

Psychoneuroimmunology

Called PNI for short, psychoneuroimmunology is a new scientific field dedicated to studying how the brain affects the immune system. In March 1982 psychologist Robert Ader and immunologist Nicholas Cohen, both of the University of Rochester, reported that, through a form of conditioning, they had caused mice to suppress their own immune systems. When the mice were given a pill they thought was an immune-suppressing drug, they reacted as if they had actually taken the drug and "directed" their bodies to turn off their immune systems.

Some scientists were skeptical that the mind could control anything as involuntary as the immune system, but Ader and Cohen's work was subsequently confirmed. Psychiatrist Malcolm Rogers and Terry Strom, an immunologist at Harvard Medical School, repeated the experiment with the same results. "We were able to condition rats to alter their immune responses," says Strom, who then took the study a step further, mixing brain chemicals with immune cells in laboratory containers. He found that some brain cells change the activity of the immune cells, but, he cautions, "We must not assume that brain chemicals mastermind immunity."

Whatever the connection, the influence is powerful. Time and again we see cases where one spouse dies and the other follows a short time later. Cause of death is usually an infectious disease that the immune system, weakened by nervous stress and grief, could not overcome.

Does this mean that we can use our brains to affect our allergies? The answer is a guarded and conditional yes. It takes special qualities to be an apt subject for mind techniques. You have to believe strongly in the brain-body connection; you have to be able to tune out the world and relax; and, most of all, you must know how to concentrate and focus your mind where you want it. If that description applies, choose a method you understand and feel comfortable with, follow its principles diligently, and let your expectations soar.

Biofeedback

This is a new technique, born in the 1960s, that teaches you to gain control of some of your involuntary physical responses. It does so by wiring you to an electronic machine that feeds back immediate body reactions *while they are happening.* You watch a monitoring device such as a meter or a screen, or listen on earphones, and note which signals you receive when you behave in certain ways.

A patient with asthma, for instance, has trouble breathing because of constricted bronchial passages. He's told to concentrate very deeply on how he feels when he's well and breathing normally. The minute he does so, his bronchial tubes get the message from the brain, begin to relax their spasms, and allow the flow of air. At the same time, he gets positive feedback in the form of a flashing light, a pattern on the screen, or a sound. When he worries or tightens up with tension, he gets a different signal. Gradually he learns which thinking processes bring positive responses and tries to master those exercises so he can utilize them when he needs them.

A 31-year-old patient was able to relieve her food allergy-addictions with dietary changes, but not her migraines. As a commercial artist, she did detailed, technical work; her ability to concentrate indicated she would make a good candidate for biofeedback.

The woman went to a recommended clinic and met a sympathetic technician who not only taught her how to use the machine but assigned "homework," with special tapes she could listen to, so that she could practice the techniques at home. She gradually learned to raise her skin temperature, which relaxed her whole body and in turn relaxed the blood vessel spasms that pressed on her brain, causing headaches. Now whenever she feels the first sign of a migraine, she stops what she's doing and concentrates on her exercises. The results have been good; she's been able to reduce both the frequency and severity of attacks.

Biofeedback is usually taught in hourly segments once a week for ten weeks; each session costs $50 or more. Some people take a few hours with a trainer or learn the basics, and then buy an inexpensive biofeedback device to train themselves at home. Once you've mastered the technique, there's no need for costly equipment. But you must continually practice and reinforce the skills you've learned or you'll lose them.

Federal Employees Health Insurance, Medicare, and Medicaid do not pay for biofeedback, but CHAMPUS, which covers the U.S. military, recently agreed to cover a wide range of biofeedback training techniques. Blue Cross, Blue Shield, and United of Omaha provide coverage in some cases; they usually ask for pre-authorization, which means you must submit the costs in advance.

Doctors say biofeedback may not work if a person has severe

pain, mental problems, or psychological stresses that prevent concentration. Motivation is also necessary. Some patients are so used to depending on medication that they can't believe they can control their symptoms themselves.

Biofeedback is not a cure. It is a technique for relaxation that has proven to be particularly effective for asthma, sinus headaches, migraines, muscle and joint pains, and as an aid to breaking food, alcohol, and drug addictions.

Hypnosis

Hypnosis can best be defined as a pathway to your unconscious mind, a state of awareness in which the conscious brain is bypassed and communication is directly established with the buried areas of your psyche.

The word *hypnosis* comes from "hypnos," Greek for sleep, and is mildly misleading. You are not asleep during hypnosis, but in a trance state, hyperaware, passive, and amenable to suggestion. A common misconception is that you lose control of your will. Ironically, you do just the opposite. By focusing all your attention and energies on a single problem, you gain control of your symptoms or emotions and learn to mobilize and direct your body's healing abilities.

In 1957 the American Medical Association recognized hypnosis as "legitimate" therapy, and since then it has become increasingly popular. Today more than 80,000 doctors, dentists, psychologists, and other professionals practice some form of hypnosis to anesthetize, psychoanalyze, and heal health problems related to tension and poor living habits.

Hypnotherapy in allergies is a growing field, with value as a stress reducer, a relaxant, and an adjunct to immunotherapy. Again, it is not a technique for weak-willed or wandering minds. The ability to concentrate is essential. Hypnosis is not something that happens to you but something that you consciously and deliberately make happen to yourself.

There are many things hypnosis will not and should not do. A Type 1 patient with mild allergies used self-hypnosis so that he could mow the lawn during pollen season. He would say to himself, "Grass is green and good for me and does not make me sneeze. I am going to go out and breathe in that wonderful, fresh-smelling pollen and I am not going to sneeze."

He claimed it worked, but one is inclined to question—perhaps he just delayed the reaction. Hypnosis should not be used to try to deceive or manipulate the body. What the patient should tell himself is: "My immune system is getting stronger and is now able to distinguish between harmless grass pollen and harmful bacteria and viruses." Rather than deliberately putting his body under stress by exposing himself to allergens, he should try to build his immune system to be able to withstand exposures over which he has no control. Hypnotherapy should help people cope with their allergic symptoms rather than be used to tell the body to turn them off.

If you're tempted to try it, don't expect immediate results, and be wary of any hypnotechnician who promises relief in a specific time. A medically trained practitioner will charge $30 and up for an hour session, individually or in a group, and will explain in advance that results can take several weeks to a year. Most medical insurance does not cover hypnosis unless performed by an M.D. But don't shop for bargains and don't go to a quack; hypnosis is too potent a tool and too easy to abuse.

One medical colleague had an experience some years ago he'll never forget. He was demonstrating the power of hypnosis to a group of residents, and a woman volunteered as a subject. He anesthetized a spot on her arm, pricked her with a needle, which she didn't feel, and woke her up. A few years later he met her at a cocktail party. During their chat she mentioned a patch of anesthesia on her arm. She had no recollection of that hypnotic episode but her unconscious was telling him about it. He realized he had never cleared that patch! He took her aside, put her into a trance, undid his work, and she was fine—much to his relief.

Few people understand how powerful hypnosis can be and that whatever you do with hypnosis you will have to undo. One should not play around with people's physical symptoms. They have a purpose: they're warning signs that something is amiss in the body. The only responsible use of hypnosis in allergies is to motivate patients to help themselves.

Hypnotherapy, then, does not have the goal of alleviating allergic symptoms, but seeks to augment or strengthen the patient's will to take positive steps, to make overdue changes in his physical environment, to start challenging himself with home testing, and to rearrange his life so that emotional stresses are minimal.

Affirmation

"Everyday, and in every way, I am becoming better and better." That statement, made by a turn-of-the-century psychotherapist named Emile Coúe, became what is ·probably the world's best-known autosuggestion. Dr. Coúe believed that if a person repeated such a thought over and over in a confident voice at times when the brain was most receptive, the idea would sink into the unconscious mind and direct behavior.

The modern version of "Coúeism" is *affirmation,* which goes one step farther by stating your desire in the present tense, as if the result has already been achieved. Instead of saying, "I am becoming better" you state, "I am better"; rather than saying, "My rash will clear up," you make a positive, definitive pronouncement: "My skin is smooth and clear."

Once you've composed your affirmation, there are many ways to implement it. You can write or type it on scraps of paper and put them around your home or office. Recite the line over and over on tape and play it to yourself when you're driving, doing chores, relaxing, or just before you go to sleep. Drum it into your head and use the affirmation to make yourself make it happen. It can't hurt you and it often helps.

Discussing this mechanism in their book, *Beyond Biofeedback,* Elmer and Alyce Green write: "The body seems to know what to do if the person knows what is desired. The body does not seem to care about the scientific accuracy of the command, or about the results per se. It simply carries out commands. Negative, destructive commands are followed, it seems, with as much success as positive commands. It is this very fact that gives rise to . . . psychosomatic diseases."

Affirmation is most effective for Type 1 patients with allergic rhinitis, sinus headaches, and skin rashes, and for such Type 2 symptoms as migraines, muscle and joint aches, and minor mental disorders. It can work for specific ailments or in a generalized way to enhance the whole immune system.

Visualization

Visualization does with mental pictures what affirmation does with words, and is especially useful as an adjunct to immunotherapy. One creative patient explains her technique: "I imagine a big pot of popcorn sitting on a burner. The kernels keep pushing up the lid and spilling out. Each one has a big red T on it. When I'm having allergic symptoms and need more T cells, I mentally turn up the heat so the flames grow larger and all these T cell kernels pop out, right into my system.

"In the lower half of the picture, lots of little B cells are lying in bed. The popcorn T cells come raining down and the B cells are unable to get up. The T cells suppress the B cells and stop my immune reaction. Amazingly, this works. One time, though, I walked into Macy's and the chemical smells hit me very fast. I tried to use visualization but I was too late. All I could conjure was a broken popcorn machine with B cells jumping all over the place.

"I learned from that," she adds. "Now I pop out more T cells *before* I go into a situation that might cause a reaction."

Visualization has several advantages. It allows you to escape into fantasy and tune out daily tensions, it can be done anywhere and any time with no special equipment, and it is private, personal, and strictly your own; you needn't share, explain, or discuss it with anyone.

Dr. Carl Simonton and his wife, Stephanie, of Fort Worth, Texas, have had great success using visualization to treat cancer. Three times a day patients listen to a tape of Dr. Simonton's voice intoning: "Take a deep breath . . . blow out . . . turn loose the tensions of the day. Feel the wave of relaxation spreading over your body. Command the muscles in your neck to relax, then the muscles across your shoulders. . . . You are allowing the tensions to flow out and more energy to flow in . . . relax more.

"Mentally picture the cancer in a way that makes sense to you. Remember the cancer cell is not powerful . . . picture your body's own white blood cells . . . see them as very strong, very aggressive, attacking the cancer cells and destroying them. See yourself beginning to feel a bit better . . . becoming more in tune with life, having more energy, a better appetite, better relationships. . . . Now at the count of three, let your eyes open up and go about your normal life."

Allergists use visualization in a similar way, stressing that patients must not think of themselves as victims of some outside force they're helpless to challenge. Allergic people have partially lost control of their immune systems. Healing involves regaining control by relearning how to discriminate between harmful agents such as viruses and bacteria and harmless agents such as dust, grass, and tree pollens.

With visualization—and indeed with all mind techniques, including Yoga, meditation, and Zen Buddhism—the degree of success depends on the depth of concentration and how skilled you are at harnessing your healing powers. Albert Schweitzer once said: "Each patient carries his own doctor inside him. They come to us not knowing that truth. We are at our best when we give the doctor who resides within each patient a chance to go to work."

BODY TECHNIQUES

These therapies depend on physical activity of some sort, be it taking vitamins, going to see a play, or climbing a mountain. Some you can do alone; others require participation of a friend, partner, or professional. Like the mind techniques, they may be useful in conjunction with medical care or, in some cases, instead of it. Unlike the mind techniques, they require little or no concentration and are probably most effective when you stop thinking about yourself and focus your thoughts and energies elsewhere.

Acupuncture

This ancient Chinese healing art treats all parts of the anatomy and every known mental or physical ailment. The theory is that your body's energy flows along imaginary lines, or meridians, that connect sensitive receptor sites beneath the skin with the internal areas of illness. These meridians have nothing to do with blood circulation or anatomical structure, and in fact make little sense to Westerners, who must take them on faith.

The technician you see should be an M.D., someone working

under medical supervision, or a person licensed by the state for independent practice. The treatment is to insert long, thin needles into body locations that correspond to—but may be very distant from—the trouble areas. Descriptions of injections vary from "a slight tingling sensation" to "extremely painful," so there's no way to predict your response. The needles stay in place twenty to thirty minutes and may or may not be preheated, twirled, or wired to electric current.

Several years ago researchers at Aberdeen University, Scotland, discovered a probable reason for the success of acupuncture: massaging specific points stimulates the pituitary gland of the brain to produce *endorphins,* morphinelike substances that relieve pain and induce a sense of well-being.

Pain relief may well explain why headaches, muscle and joint aches, and abdominal cramps are among the allergic conditions frequently improved by acupuncture. But asthma, hay fever, and cerebral disorders get better as well, perhaps as a result of endorphin euphoria or of other body reactions that are still a mystery. Dr. Michael O. Smith, a psychiatrist at Lincoln Hospital in New York, notes that acupuncture "has been known to boost white blood count and stabilize hormone levels," which may (1) indicate some strengthening of the immune system and (2) explain the alleviation of allergic symptoms caused by hormone imbalance.

Disadvantages of this therapy are that relief is short-term and that treatments may produce discomfort, can be costly ($350 and up for ten sessions), and eliminate symptoms rather than causes. Some insurance companies cover acupuncture, realizing that it might be less expensive than alternative treatments or surgery. Other firms honor claims only when a physician does the needling. Medicaid, Medicare, and most Blue Cross plans don't provide coverage at all.

The greatest advantage of acupuncture is that it works.

Acupressure

Acupressure can work, too, mainly for allergic headaches. The name is newer than the technique: a strong finger pressure applied to any of 102 specific contact points on the body. Some call it "needle-free acupuncture," or use the Japanese term *shiatsu.* The joy of this method is that you can do it yourself at home; no appointment or special tools are necessary.

To find one of the basic headache locations, drop your chin to your chest, and probe the back of your neck for two indentations at the base of your skull. When you feel them, push up against the skull bone until you hit sensitive spots on either side. Press the spots or the area (if you can't find the spots) as hard as you can for thirty seconds. If you notice relief, you may want to develop the technique further. Most chiropractors can instruct you in acupressure, and many colleges and university extensions teach it in classes.

A word of warning: Beware of ads peddling "acupressure wrist bands" that are "guaranteed to reduce gastrointestinal symptoms." The only thing they'll reduce is your bank account.

Chiropractic

The science of chiropractic maintains that readjusting the spinal column can help the body control such allergic symptoms as headaches, fatigue, muscle spasms, asthma, and just about everything else. The theory is that misaligned vertebrae obstruct the flow of nerve energy and cause sympathetic reactions in different parts of the body. When the vertebrae are realigned, the obstructions are removed, nerve energy flows as it should, and natural healing forces go back to work.

Chiropractors who work in conjunction with physicians can often be effective because of the strong connection between nerves and allergy. In experiments with rabbits, scientists have been able to stop an asthmatic bronchial spasm by cutting the nerve from the bronchial tube to the brain. Chiropractors feel they can achieve similar results by manipulating the spine and redirecting nerve energy.

Chiropractic treatment starts with a careful examination of the neck and spine to determine the nature and extent of misalignment. The practitioner then makes an *adjustment,* a rapid, sudden movement applying force to a specific point in the vertebra. This is done to remove nerve interference and realign structure.

The patient usually gets one or two adjustments a week for ten weeks, and then once a month as preventive treatment. Each session costs from $8 to $25 and is covered by most types of medical insurance. Chiropractors often suggest long-term commitment to therapy "to help preserve health and avoid the pain, disability, and cost of ill health." Some patients balk at the necessity for continuing treatment indefinitely; others believe in a lifelong maintenance program and go along with it.

Stress Reduction

"The relationship of stress and behavior to cardiovascular conditions is well documented," says C. David Jenkins, Ph.D., medical professor at the University of Texas in Galveston. What is not widely known is . . . its ability to depress the body's immune system."

Scientists generally agree that conquering stress allows the immune system to grow stronger, regain efficient functioning, and avoid the T cell degeneration that leads to the development of allergies. Patients can aid this process by seeking activities that take their minds off themselves and their daily woes.

Some possibilities might include the following: learning to play an instrument, speak a foreign language, or paint a watercolor; going to see a movie, taking a friend to lunch, visiting an outdoor flea market, getting a massage, or giving one to someone you love. Do anything but sit around and mope. You'lll find that allergic symptoms which are bothersome but manageable take a back seat to any activity commanding your attention and your energies.

Sex Therapy

Some patients report that their symptoms clear, almost miraculously, during and after sexual intercourse. This is not imagination. Granted, the sex act generally takes your mind off your allergies and elevates your mood, but there's a physiological reason for feeling better, too. Sex stimulates the flow of adrenalin, also known as epinephrine, the hormone that the adrenal glands secrete in times of stress and that enables a 130-pound woman to lift a two-ton car off her trapped child.

Adrenalin also relaxes bronchial tissue and raises blood pressure, increasing the flow of blood from the head and decongesting the nasal passages. Type 1 persons are often amazed to hear themselves say, after intercourse, "Hey, I can breathe again!" Unfortunately, such beneficial effects are short-term, although they possibly last longer for Type 2 persons.

"Sex for me will totally stop a reaction for several days," says a Type 2 woman patient. "When I was really sick, having severe reactions all the time, and when nothing else helped, I could always count on sex. Maybe it was the release of adrenalin, or maybe, because I was having cerebral symptoms and feeling isolated, it was the closeness and the idea that someone cared about me."

There can be negative reactions as well. Asthmatics sometimes find that heavy breathing aggravates wheezing. Increased body heat may change a lover's soap, cologne, or deodorant into irritating gases. And contraceptives may be potent allergens. Dr. H. L. Newbold, author of *Dr. Newbold's Revolutionary New Discoveries About Weight Loss*, reports the following: "I had one woman—who turned out to be allergic to the spermicide used on her diaphragm—who felt a compelling desire to go on an eating spree while having intercourse. She would then lose all interest in sex, fake great passion and multiple orgasms so her partner would hurry and finish. Then she'd jump out of bed and make for the kitchen."

An August 1982 *Newsweek* article tells of a woman who developed hives after intercourse. Lab tests confirmed that she was allergic to semen, although she had thought her reaction was part of an orgasm. The hives disappeared when her lover began using condoms.

More commonly, people react to materials on their partners' clothing, hair, and skin, especially cat and dog hairs, perfume, and tobacco smoke. There have been many cases where partners could not understand why their symptoms erupted during sex. A woman who is allergic to horses but lives with a jockey, a man who is sensitive to ink and married to a graphic artist, a Type 2 man in love with a woman who sells cosmetics—all will have problems during intimacy. The "contaminated" partner can prevent such complications by wearing protective clothing while working, taking it off before entering the house (impractical but not impossible), and showering before intercourse.

Both partners should be encouraged to endure minor inconveniences and make concessions. People with happy personal relationships live longer and are more capable of coping with immune system malfunctions than people who add domestic woes to their pile of stresses.

Monogamy is strongly urged for the allergic person. The reasons have nothing to do with morality, religion, ethical commitments, or sexual preferences. But Mother Nature is telling us something with all these new diseases such as genital herpes and AIDS (Acquired Immune Deficiency Syndrome), an affliction seen mainly in male homosexuals, in which the body loses its ability to fight off infections and often develops Kaposi's sarcoma, a rare, virulent form of skin cancer. Both AIDS and herpes have reached epidemic proportions in the United States over the past two years.

There are sound biological reasons for monogamy. People with many sexual exposures have immune systems that are severely crippled from battling bacteria, and are therefore much more susceptible to allergic reactions. Not only do various partners bring pollens, animal dander, and chemicals from their workplaces into bed, they also bring body fluids such as semen, with its high concentration of foreign antigens.

The same thing happens both in homosexual and heterosexual intercourse; two people are exchanging vast amounts of these antigens. Multiple exposures may have the same immunologic consequences as multiple blood transfusions from different donors. Compound the sites of sexual activity to include oral and rectal, and you greatly increase the chance of transmitting hostile viruses and breaking down the immune system. Allergic men who are not monogamous should use condoms during intercourse, and allergic women, unless they're monogamous, should urge their partners to do so.

Problems may be complicated by use of the birth-control pill. Despite copious data, little is known about its long-term effects. A number of women get their first allergic symptom after starting the pill, and there is a close correlation with migraines.

Nevertheless, a regular, monogamous sex life is one of the best possible treatments for allergies. Enjoy it with someone you love as often as you can. It not only makes you feel better, but it's also a great motivator to take the steps you should take to get back to health.

Exercise

Another activity that's good for almost everyone's health is exercise. Whether or not you should partake depends on the specific activity, your own sensitivities, your allergic state of health at the time, and how strenuously you indulge. Exercise relieves some allergies and exacerbates others.

In most cases, common sense will dictate your behavior. If you're a Type 1 with respiratory problems, you'll want to avoid outdoor workouts in cool weather, as breathing in cold, dry air at a rapid rate is almost certain to bring on symptoms. Wearing a mask or kerchief over your mouth and nose allows you to warm and moisten the air before it reaches your nasal passages and lungs, but it may cause more embarrassment than it's worth.

Type 1 persons can often benefit from moderate, noncompetitive activities such as dancing or exercising indoors, hiking in the mountains, walking or bicycling in clear, fresh air, and swimming in heated water without submerging their heads.

The same good sense should keep you far away from swimming pools if you're a chlorine-sensitive Type 2. Nor should you walk, jog, or run in polluted areas or on smoggy days. Gyms with well-oiled or new plastic equipment, mechanical bowling alleys, and tennis courts with chemical-composition floors can also bother you, as can spectator sports if you attend such events as auto races, which generate great quantities of dirt, dust, and exhaust fumes.

Yet many Type 2 patients find that exercise is a remarkably effective way to burn off a bad reaction. One young man who knows he must occasionally go to his boss's home for dinner, where he will have to endure the fumes from gas heating, always leaves the next morning free for hiking or "running it off" in the fresh country air.

Dr. Jordan Fink at the Medical College of Wisconsin in Milwaukee warns, however, that exercise can be potentially deadly if it follows eating a food to which you're allergic. He treated a patient for anaphylactic shock simply because she had nibbled celery before a dance class. There seems to be a synergistic reaction greater than that which would normally be expected, so if you must eat an allergenic food, stay quiet for several hours afterward.

Similar advice comes from two Harvard physicians, K. Frank

Austen and Albert L. Sheffer, who claim that exercising too soon after eating can cause "exercise allergy," an unusual condition that affects athletes after periods of prolonged exertion. The symptoms are bronchospasm and labored breathing, extremely itchy hives, stomach cramps, palpitations, and a dramatic drop in blood pressure that sometimes leads to unconsciousness. Drs. Austen and Sheffer draw no conclusions, but warn that this syndrome can be a real threat to athletes who have a personal or family history of allergy. They advise possible subjects to work out with a friend and to carry injectable adrenalin.

The safest approach is to experiment and see what kind of exercise makes you feel best. The increased blood circulation and oxygen intake will stimulate your energies and keep you physically and emotionally alert, and in some cases will provide definite relief of symptoms.

Vitamins

So many outrageous claims have been made for vitamin and megavitamin therapy that it's often difficult to separate the quacks and hucksters from the responsible scientists. Although the latter have reached numerous conclusions that have been thoroughly researched and found to be accurate, the conventional medical establishment has never felt there was sufficient evidence to recommend vitamins. The Food and Drug Administration's present position, in fact, is that "Taking excess vitamins is a complete waste, both in money and effect. Anyone who eats a reasonably varied diet of whole food should normally never need vitamins."

A number of doctors would disagree, particularly those who practice *orthomolecular,* or megavitamin, therapy, which advocates good nutrition and the use of vitamins, minerals, and other natural body substances to restore homeostasis—inner body balance. At the same time, these physicians warn that vitamin overdose (particularly A and D) can be harmful.

Other doctors claim preventive qualities. Lendon Smith, M.D., author of *Foods for Healthy Kids,* states that "If vitamin C (500 to 2,000 mg), calcium (500 to 1,000 mg), and B_6 (100 mg) are given to a victim of allergy 30 to 60 minutes prior to his exposure to the offending substance, he will not have an allergic response." Would it were that easy.

The wisest course is moderation in the form of a daily vitamin-and-mineral tablet taken with a meal (if there's no food to absorb the nutrients, they pass through the body without being utilized). Obviously, patients allergic to any of the fillers and binders in vitamins, such as sugar, dyes, corn, alfalfa, or yeast, should refrain. Type 2 patients who react to traces of the petrochemicals used to make synthetic vitamins may do better with natural ones, even though the molecular structure is exactly the same. All drugstores and health-food stores carry natural vitamins, but be sure to ask what's in them, and if the salesperson doesn't know, don't buy them. Write to the company first or order from a firm that lists all ingredients on their labels.

Very new evidence shows that vitamins B and C disappear more rapidly from the blood of animals exposed to oxidizing air pollutants such as ozone, and suggests that Type 2 persons might benefit from increased supplements on smoggy days.

In general, vitamin C seems valuable to all allergic patients for its antihistamine and immune-boosting qualities; vitamin A helps build respiratory tissue and resistance to infection; topical E aids the healing of some skin rashes; B-complex vitamins produce antibodies and regenerate blood cells; and the rest, in small quantities, probably won't hurt you. The next five years should reveal a great deal more about how and why vitamins work and what role they will play, if any, in some of the amazing new allergy tests and treatments now being developed.

Chapter 7
WHAT'S IN THE FUTURE

Whoever said "The future lies ahead" was not only redundant but inaccurate. The future is here. Much that has been researched, discussed, and predicted is beginning to materialize. New theories are becoming obsolete before they're even accepted.

Within the next few years improved laboratory techniques will make Type 1 testing a matter of taking a blood sample and determining from it exactly what substances cause reactions and the correct dosages for treatment.

Scientists are hoping to develop blood tests for Type 2 cerebral disorders as well, and have in fact spent twenty years trying to discover exactly which blood component carries the evidence. New research suggests that the level of a chemical called DOPEG (3,4-dihydroxyphenylglycol) appears to be higher in biologically depressed people. Patients who improved after taking an antidepressant drug showed a significant decrease in DOPEG levels.

Such experiments, it is hoped, will eventually lead to standardized tests for cerebral allergies. Also, as more and more evidence proves that erratic behavior can be caused by the action of chemicals on the brain, the stigma of mental illness will diminish.

More precise and effective immunotherapy for both Type 1 and Type 2 patients will be possible as the commercial firms that prepare antigen extracts gain standardization and turn out uniform products that can be replaced and reproduced. New techniques will allow doctors to immunize people more rapidly and to many more substances. In 1980, for example, Dr. Timothy J. Sullivan of Dallas reported that he and two other doctors experimented with thirty penicillin-allergic people. The subjects were able to tolerate a normal penicillin injection after a speeded-up desensitization process that took only four hours.

Avoidance will be less of a problem for Type 1 patients as hypersensitive instruments help us to predict pollen areas and seasons; Type 2 persons can look forward to the utilization of new energy sources so that homes and buildings will no longer have to be sealed off from pollution. Levels of formaldehyde and other toxic substances in the air will decline as industry produces safe substitutes. Public awareness will force reduced exposure to tobacco smoke and strong scents, and nontoxic living will become an accepted reality rather than an uphill battle.

THERAPIES TO COME

New drugs, new theories, and new therapies will be available to prevent, alleviate, and stop allergic reactions. Some look very promising.

Bone Marrow Transplantation

This technique goes one step further than transfer factor, the substance that transfers immunities from donor to recipient. Immune cells grow in the bone marrow, and it is now possible to transplant the whole "garden." The procedure is not difficult: multiple aspirations (suction through needles) are performed under general anesthesia. The substance is carefully filtered and processed, and then injected intravenously. Transfer factor stimulates the recipient's T cells to function; bone marrow transplant actually puts the donor's T cells into the recipient's blood. So instead of tuning the car's engine, you'll be replacing it with a new engine.

At present, however, the drawbacks are serious. The recipient must be carefully matched with an identical donor, usually a sibling, and the chances of a sibling's being suitable are only one in four. Strong drugs and radiation must be given to turn off the patient's own immune system so that he accepts the transplant. In spite of these precautions, the patient may develop graft-versus-host disease (rejection), with symptoms of fever, dermatitis, hepatitis, pneumonia, alopecia (loss of hair), diarrhea, and increased susceptibility to infection.

Nevertheless, researchers are working on ways to refine bone marrow transplantation to reduce the odds of serious side effects. When they do, probably within the next five years, the result will be an injectable serum that provides resistance to allergies for twelve months to a lifetime.

Brain Repair

Some Type 2 allergies can cause convulsive seizures and other cerebral reactions severe enough to damage brain cell tissue. At the University of Lund in Sweden, neurologist Anders Bjorklund has been able to successfully graft neurons (brain cells) and change the behavior of brain-damaged rats.

Scientists feel that brain cell grafts will be available for humans in the next decade. Fifty years of evidence indicates that the brain is immunologically tolerant; transplants will be rejected, if at all, at a much slower rate than at other body sites. Also, there will be less need to match brain tissue genetically than is necessary for other body tissues.

Very different experiments at the University of California in Irvine show that brain injuries trigger the release of healing chemicals called *neuronotrophic factors*. Psychobiologist Carl Cotman predicts that we will one day be able to produce neuronotrophic factors through genetic engineering, feed them back to persons with brain tissue damage, and thus augment the body's own processes.

Severely allergic Type 2 patients and universal reactors who had no hopes of recovering from cerebral injuries now have cause for optimism. We are entering an exciting era of brain repair.

Monoclonal Antibodies

The term simply refers to a hybrid cell with two main characteristics: it can produce antibodies, a capacity it gets from a B cell, and it can reproduce itself endlessly, an ability it takes from a cancer cell. The result is a kind of super antibody-producing cell that's able to make limitless supplies of identical selves, or *clones*, outside the body in a laboratory.

For years scientists have been looking for a way to reproduce large amounts of very pure antibodies for test and research purposes. Now they have one, and they're beginning to use *monoclonal antibodies* in several areas of immunological research. For the first time scientists can study the antigen-antibody reaction at the chemical level.

More important is the future possibility that a monoclonal antibody can be produced to be injected into the bloodstream of allergic patients. There it would give the body a supply of specific immune proteins that would prevent allergic reactions. The technology is still in its infancy, but many companies are researching ways to convert this discovery into testing and treatment procedures for cancer, leukemia, and other diseases as well. The FDA estimates that the market for products containing monoclonal antibodies will reach the billion-dollar range in the current decade.

Antiidiotypic Antibodies

An *idiotype*, in this sense, refers to the specific antibody that causes an allergic reaction. An *antiidiotypic antibody* (AIA) is an antibody directed against the symptom-causing antibody, like an antimissile missile.

The AIA is not a drug but a protein synthesized from actual body cells. It won't cause any of the side effects associated with drug use. Cells have a way of telling each other to stop a reaction, and researchers have been able to isolate the chemicals that contain this message. When injected back into the body, they can stop both Type 1 and Type 2 reactions, and the effect of a single shot will last six months.

AIAs are among the most promising of all the new treatments being researched. They should be sufficiently tested and refined to be available to the public in five to seven years.

Gene Therapy

Very new research has identified the exact region of the B cell that contains the genes that determine your specific allergic sensitivities. Scientists are seeking ways to release these genes and make their genetic information available for laboratory alteration.

Many obstacles lie in the path of the ultimate goal of introducing a "therapeutic" gene into the human embryo, or into body tissue of a newborn baby whose immune rejection system is not yet fully developed, in order to have that gene correct inherited weaknesses and provide specific immunities. Nor is there any way to ensure that these laboratory-produced genes will function as intended.

One researcher, Bob Williamson of St. Mary's Hospital Medical School in London, reports: "Gene therapy is not yet possible, but may become feasible soon, particularly for well-understood gene defects. We may be able to alter the individual's inheritance as well as the way his body works. In my view . . . knowledge of the genetic factors is more likely to lead to new pharmacological approaches, and to prevention, than gene therapy."

Others are convinced that in the next fifteen to twenty years scientists will be able to manufacture an injectable gene that will provide specific or nonspecific body immunity, and thus eliminate allergic reactions in the recipients and in all their heirs.

What Else Is New?

The allergy sweepstakes race is on, but the prize won't go to one person alone. The accumulated research of thousands of dedicated scientists will one day evolve into the safest and most effective therapy yet discovered. And even though the person who makes the last discovery may reap the glory, the medical world will know the truth: the combined and determined efforts of many will have made the ultimate breakthrough possible.

What will it be? It could be any of the preceding therapies or perhaps one of the following. Research at the Johns Hopkins Allergic Diseases Center in Baltimore centers around biweekly shots of a "conjugated allergen," a stepped-up desensitization process that appears to be safer and faster than conventional injections for Type 1 inhalants. It is still in the experimental stages.

Other experiments at Johns Hopkins are pursuing a way of desensitizing people against pollen antigen through the nose rather than the bloodstream, or by injecting a new kind of steroid—one that has minimal side effects—directly into the nose. Drs. Kimishige and Teruko Ishizaka have identified substances in rat tissue that raise and lower IgE levels, which can produce or eliminate allergy. They are looking for a way to stop the cells from producing IgE molecules against harmless antigens and thus end all Type 1 allergies once and for all.

Scientists are working on Type 2 allergies in quieter and less publicized ways, but with equal diligence. One experiment concerns rheumatoid arthritis, an autoimmune (when the body makes antibodies against its own tissues) disorder that often accompanies and results from Type 2 allergies. Studies at the University of Miami in Florida have shown that daily injections, for fourteen days, of the venom of a Bolivian ant causes a two- to three-year remission in some patients. Researchers are continuing their work and awaiting FDA approval.

It would take another book to list all the experiments in progress. No one can predict which of the hundreds of theories now being researched will fade into obscurity or which will make medical history and endure. The important fact is that a great many people are trying.

FEWER PRESCRIPTION DRUGS

Another reason for optimism is that Americans are using far fewer drugs in the 1980s than they did in the late 1970s, according to a study recently completed by the National Institute of Mental Health. Sales of Valium and sleeping pills dropped by over 50 percent, and prescriptions for all drugs declined by 7 percent, even though there were more than ever on the market. A NIMH official commented that "Americans have become aware that there are risks and benefits to be weighed in drug taking. They are starting to ask about all possible effects of a prescription drug, and in fact if they truly need to take it."

The trend to question the need for taking prescription drugs seems to be increasing. A recent study at Johns Hopkins Hospital found in a random survey that "patients who did not receive prescriptions reported more satisfaction with the communicative aspects of their visits to physicians than patients who did receive prescriptions. The physician who gives verbal attention to the patient's problem by taking time to understand and answer questions, give explanations, and show a friendly interest in the patient has a satisfying effect, and may have a psychologically therapeutic effect on that patient."

"Prescriptions," concluded the report in the December 1981

issue of the *American Journal of Public Health,* "sometimes may be used as a poor substitute for 'meaningful' interaction during the visit and serve as a kind of shortcut in the medical care process."

Along with the trend to use fewer prescription drugs, scientists are seeking ways to reduce drug potency. One approach has been suggested by Drs. Robert Ader and Nicholas Cohen of Rochester University. Their research into the way placebos work convinced them that not only can people be conditioned to think they're getting a drug when they're not, but they can also be conditioned to think they're getting full medication when the dosage has been halved. The obvious advantage will be to reduce drug dependency and side effects while still giving the patient complete therapeutic benefits.

The field of *pharmacokinetics* may revolutionize drug therapy in a different way. Pharmacokinetics is the study of how drugs react in the body after they're swallowed, injected, or absorbed. Responses are measured by testing the amount of medication in the individual's urine, blood, and tissues to determine how the body assimilates the substance. From those figures, a doctor can calculate the minimum dose needed for a drug to perform its function. Since each person's tolerance and sensitivities are different, it may take three pills to do for one person what half a tablet does for another.

This could be a remarkable tool. If there were a simple blood test to determine each person's minimum dose, scientists believe we could cut down our intake of medication and drugs by 50 percent or more. One thing is certain: drugs of the future will be based on natural body chemicals produced in laboratories with the help of genetically engineered blood cells and body fluids. These new medications will be less addictive and have fewer side effects, and their goal will be to enhance the body's own production of healing substances rather than to take their place.

NO MORE ALLERGIES

A growing number of scientists feel that the next decade will bring a realization that the words "allergy" and "immune system" are both obsolete. The word allergy was coined by a pediatrician who was studying hay fever, and means "altered or abnormal reaction." Immune derives from the Latin for "exempt from costs or taxation" and referred to the way animals and humans exempted themselves from the costs of disease. Both words are too limiting to describe the functions they deal with.

There will be no more allergies by the year 2000 because the concept of what allergies are will no longer be valid. What we now know of as Type 1 and Type 2 symptoms will not be seen as separate functions of a single immune network but as a part of a *regulatory system*—a vast umbrella that covers the neurological (nervous) and endocrine (glandular) systems as well.

Some doctors speak of this as a trend toward "lumpology"— lumping together the three systems: immune, neurological, and endocrine—and are merging treatments accordingly.

At the patient level, it means that diabetes will no longer be considered solely a glandular disorder, hay fever will not be considered an "abnormal reaction" to pollens, and psychiatric disease will not be considered a behavioral disorder mainly caused by situational stresses. Instead, patients will visit a *regulatory specialist* who will consider their symptoms in terms of an altered homeostasis—that is, an imbalance of body mechanisms. The physician will investigate the imbalance and attempt to adjust it in order to bring the body back to homeostasis.

Today a person with multiple sclerosis and hay fever probably sees a neurologist for treatment of the former and an allergist for the latter, and most likely neither doctor consults the other. Yet you wouldn't think of having one mechanic work on the transmission of your car and a second person fix the valves without telling each what the other is doing. Better yet, you'd have one skilled mechanic do both jobs. In much the same way, the current tendency to specialize in medicine will be reversed as doctors find themselves becoming "systems supervisors" rather than "parts mechanics."

When the three major specialties coalesce into one another, it will no longer be scientifically accurate to say that a disease is associated with only one organ system. This consolidation will give doctors a broader and more complete picture of what's happening in the patient's body as well as suggesting many more possible avenues of treatment. It will offer allergy and other patients renewed hope that, by fine-tuning their bodies' inner mechanisms, they will achieve a return to health that is both in accordance with nature and long-lasting.

Meanwhile, research on all fronts continues assiduously. Scientists maintain that within the next few decades they will find the key to switch off the pathologic mechanisms that cause pain and illness, thus assuring lives that are free both of drugs and of symptoms. The pieces of the great biological puzzle known as allergy are gradually coming together.

GLOSSARY

Additive: Any substance added to a food to produce a desired effect.

Adrenalin: See *epinephrine*.

Affirmation: The act of making a positive statement and repeating it over and over in an attempt to enhance healing.

Alkali salts: A mixture of soluble salts (sodium, potassium, and calcium bicarbonate) that helps neutralize body acids produced in an allergic reaction.

Allergen: A substance that causes an allergic reaction; an antigen.

Allergenic: Causing or producing an allergic reaction.

Allergic rhinitis: Seasonal or perennial nasal inflammation.

Allergy: An abnormal response to a substance well tolerated by most people.

Anaphylactic shock: A severe allergic reaction, characterized by vomiting, cramps, and swollen throat passages, that makes breathing difficult; suffocation and death may follow.

Anaphylaxis: An extreme and immediate allergic reaction.

Angioedema: Giant hives usually accompanied by swelling.

Antibody: A protein molecule produced to fight off and protect the body from foreign substances.

Antigen: Any substance that causes the body to produce antibodies.

Antihistamine: A drug that counteracts the effects of histamine and stops or prevents allergic reactions.

Appestat: The appetite control center in the brain.

Applied kinesiology: The testing of muscle strength before and after exposure to an allergen. Weakened muscle power is said to indicate a positive reaction.

Aroma therapy: Using natural plant essences or chemical odors to affect physical and emotional responses.

Asthma: A condition caused by an obstruction of the bronchial tubes that is usually allergic and produces coughing, wheezing, shortness of breath, and chest constriction.

Autogenous: Originating or derived from sources within the same individual, such as an autogenous skin graft.

Autoimmune: A condition produced when the body makes antibodies against its own tissues or fluids.

Avoidance: The best treatment for allergies; the clearing away of allergenic substances.

B cells: White blood cells that produce antibodies.

Biofeedback: The technique of making involuntary bodily processes perceptible in order to manipulate them by conscious control.

Biological food families: A system for classifying foods based on similar appearance and anatomical structure.

Bronchitis: Inflammation of the bronchial tubes or air passages in the lungs.

Candida albicans: A genus of yeastlike fungi normally found in the body but which can multiply and cause infections or allergic sensitivity.

Candidiasis: Yeast disease; an infection caused by an overgrowth of the yeastlike fungi that are part of the normal flora of the mouth, skin, intestinal tract, and vagina.

Cerebral allergy: Mental disorders caused by sensitivity to foods or synthetic chemicals in the environment.

Chemotherapy: The use of drugs or medication in the treatment or control of disease.

Chiropractic: A system for adjusting misalignments of the spine to correct the cause of disease.

Clinical ecology: A new branch of medicine that treats both Type 1 and Type 2 allergies through diet and environmental control, and preferably without the use of drugs.

Contact dermatitis: A skin rash resulting from touching an allergen.

Contactant: An allergen capable of inducing skin sensitivity after being touched one or more times.

Cytotoxic test: A blood test purporting to determine food and chemical allergies by noting the action of a specific antigen on the patient's white blood cells.

Dander: Tiny particles from skin, feathers, or hair of an animal, which frequently cause allergies.

Desensitization: The process of building up the body's tolerance to allergens by injections of sublingual drops of dilutions of the allergenic substances.

Dilution: A fluid that has been diluted or made less potent.

Diuretic: A medication to increase the flow of urine.

Ecology unit: A diagnostic hospital run by clinical ecologists for severely allergic Type 2 patients and universal reactors.

Eczema: A dry, itchy skin rash caused by allergy.

Edema: A swelling of body tissues due to accumulation of fluids.

Elimination diet: A diet devoid of commonly allergenic foods and those suspected of causing allergic symptoms in a specific patient.

Endorphins: Morphinelike substances produced by the brain and said to relieve pain and induce a sense of well-being.

Eosinophils: White blood cells that, in increased numbers, indicate the presence of Type 1 allergy.

Ephinephrine: A powerful hormone that relaxes bronchial spasms, raises blood pressure, and is necessary for treating anaphylactic shock; trade name Adrenalin.

Ergotamines: A class of ergot-derived drugs that constrict blood vessels and help control migraines.

FDA: The Food and Drug Administration, a government regulatory agency.

Food addiction: An allergic reaction similar to drug addiction; the person becomes hooked on a particular food and must keep eating it in order not to experience withdrawal symptoms.

Formaldehyde: A colorless, irritating gas used chiefly as a disinfectant and preservative and in synthesizing other compounds.

Gastrointestinal: Relating to both stomach and intestines.

Glucose: A simple sugar that is easily absorbed into the body metabolism.

Hay fever: Seasonal rhinitis caused mainly by pollens.

Histamine: A body substance, released in allergic reactions, that causes symptoms.

Homeostasis: Internal balance; a tendency to stability in the normal physiological state of the organism; good health.

House dust mites: Microscopic creatures that live in house dust; their carcasses and excrement are potent allergens.

Hypersensitivity: The allergic state.

Hyposensitization: See *desensitization*.

Immune system: The mechanism by which the body recognizes materials as foreign to itself and has the power to neutralize, metabolize, or eliminate.

Immunity: The state of being able to resist a particular antigen by producing antibodies to counteract it.

Immunoglobulin: A specific antibody.

Immunotherapy: Stimulation of the immune system for the purpose of treating allergies and other illnesses.

Immunotoxic: Pertaining to chemicals that do the greatest damage to the immune system.

Inhalant: Any airborne substance tiny enough to be inhaled into the lungs.

Intradermal test: An allergy test performed by injecting antigen into the skin and measuring the wheal it provokes.

Irritant: An agent that produces local inflammation.

Kaposi's sarcoma: A rare, virulent form of skin cancer seen mainly in male homosexuals.

Mast cells: Large cells containing histamine, found in the mucous membranes, bronchial tubes, and skin; cells where Type 1 allergic reactions occur.

Migraine: A condition marked by recurrent severe headaches, often accompanied by nausea and vomiting and frequently attributed to food allergy.

Mold: A superficial growth of fungus that produces tiny, lightweight airborne spores.

Mucous membranes: Moist tissue that forms the lining of body cavities which have an external opening, such as the nasal and digestive tracts.

Nasal polyps: Fluid-filled growths in the nose that frequently block the nasal passages and are sometimes related to allergies.

Neutralize: To render an allergic reaction inactive.

Nonspecific therapy: Allergy treatment directed toward building up the immune system as a whole.

Nystatin: An antifungal antibiotic that selectively attacks *Candida albicans*.

Organic foods: Foods grown without chemical fertilizers or pesticides.

Orthomolecular: Pertaining to therapy that advocates good nutrition and the use of vitamins, minerals, and other natural body substances to restore health.

Petrochemical: A synthetic chemical derived from petroleum or natural gas.

Pharmacokinetics: The study of how the body absorbs, metabolizes, distributes, and excretes drugs.

Placebo: An inert or innocuous substance containing no drugs, used to provide mental relief or, in controlled experiments, to test the efficacy of a drug.

Pollen: The microscopic seeds of trees, grasses, and flowers that form a fine, airborne dust and can cause allergic reactions.

Pollutant: Any substance that makes something unclean.

Postnasal drip: A condition in which nasal fluids leak down into the back of the pharynx, often causing a sore throat.

Propanolol: A new drug used mainly to reduce blood pressure and touted as a migraine preventive: trade name Inderal.

Provocative-Neutralization (P-N) Test: An allergy test that uses an antigen to provoke a reaction and then neutralizes the reaction with a lower dose of the same antigen that provoked it.

Pruritis: Itching.

Psychoneuroimmunology (PNI): A new science that links the brain and the immune system.

Pulse test: A test, developed by Dr. Arthur Coca, that involves taking the pulse before and after exposure to an allergen. If the pulse rises, the substance is said to be allergenic.

RAST (radioallergosorbent test): A blood test for Type 1 allergies.

Respiratory tract: The system that starts at the nostrils, runs through the nose to the back of the throat, and then down into the larynx and lungs.

Rhinitis: Inflammation of the mucous membrane of the nose; a nasal condition accompanied by sneezing, congestion, and the discharge of watery fluid.

Rotation diet: A diet in which a particular food is eaten only once every four or five days.

Scratch test: A test in which a specific antigen is scratched onto the skin; if the body is sensitive, a red, itchy wheal develops.

Sensitization: The process that leads to the development of allergic symptoms in persons intolerant of a specific substance.

Serum: In allergy, the desensitizing liquid or antigens.

Sodium cromolyn: An inhalant medication used to prevent allergic responses, especially asthmatic bronchial spasms; trade name Intal.

Specific therapy: Allergy treatment directed towards a particular antigen.

Steroids: Synthetic compounds used in severe allergic cases to suppress the action of the immune system.

Sublingual: Under the tongue.

Sublingual drops: An antigen squirted under the tongue to diagnose or neutralize an allergic reaction and to effect desensitivity.

Synergism: The action of two or more substances to produce an effect that neither could achieve alone.

Synthetic: Made in a laboratory; not produced normally in nature.

T cells: White blood cells that direct B cells to produce antibodies in an allergic reaction.

Tolerance threshold: The maximum amount of allergens a person can endure without reacting.

Transfer factor: An extract of white blood cells that transfers immunities from donor to recipient.

Type 1: A person mainly allergic to pollens, dust, animal dander, and molds and who usually reacts with respiratory symptoms.

Type 2: A person mainly allergic to foods and synthetic chemicals in the environment and who reacts with cerebral and other symptoms.

Tyramine: An organic substance found in certain foods that is capable of swelling blood vessels and is said to cause migraines.

Universal reactor: A person allergic to almost everything.

Urticaria: Allergic hives or welts.

Urushiol: The irritating oil of the sap of poison oak and poison ivy that causes an itchy skin rash.

Vascular: Pertaining to blood vessels.

Visualization: The act of forming mental images and using them to enhance healing and reduce allergic and other symptoms.

Wheal: A sudden elevation of the skin surface that is measured to determine the degree of allergic reactivity.

Withdrawal: The unpleasant group of symptoms associated with the removal of a food to which a person is addicted.

Appendix 1

BIOLOGICAL FOOD FAMILIES

PLANTS

Algae family
  agar agar
  carrageen (Irish moss)
  dulse
  kelp (seaweed)
Arrowroot family
  arrowroot (Maranta starch)
Arum family
  arrowroot (colocasia)
  poi
  taro arrowroot
Banana family
  arrowroot (Musa)
  banana
  plantain
Beech family
  beechnut
  chestnut
Birch family
  filbert (hazelnut)
  wintergreen
Borage family
  borage
  comfrey
Buckwheat family
  buckwheat

honey, buckwheat
rhubarb
Buttercup family
  golden seal
Cactus
  prickly pear
Canna family
  arrowroot, Queensland
Caper family
  caper
Carpetweed family
  New Zealand spinach
Carrot family
  angelica
  anise
  caraway seed
  carrot
  celeriac
  celery
  chervil
  coriander
  cumin
  dill
  fennel
  lovage
  parsley
  parsnip
Cashew family

cashew
mango
pistachio
Citrus family
  citron
  grapefruit
  honey
    grapefruit
    lemon blossom
    lime
    orange blossom
  kumquat
  lemon
  lime
  orange
  tangelo
  tangerine
Composite family
  artichoke
  chamomile
  chicory
  dandelion
  endive
  escarole
  honey
    safflower
    star thistle
  goldenrod
  Jerusalem artichoke
  lettuce
  safflower oil
  salsify
  sunflower seeds
  tarragon
  yarrow
Conifer family
  honey, conifer
  juniper (gin)
  pine nut
Cycad family
  Florida arrowroot (Zamia)
  Dillenia family

kiwi berry
Dogwood family
  honey, tupelo
Ebony family
  persimmon
Eucalyptus family
  honey, eucalyptus
Flax family
  flaxseed
Fungi family
  baker's yeast
  brewer's or nutritional yeast
  mushroom
  truffle
Ginger family
  arrowroot, East Indian
    (Curcuma)
  cardamon
  ginger
  turmeric
Ginseng family
  ginseng
Goosefoot family
  beet
  chard
  lamb's quarters
  spinach
  sugar beet
Gourd family
  cantaloupe
  casaba melon
  crenshaw melon
  chayote
  Chinese preserving melon
  cucumber
  honeydew melon
  muskmelon
  Persian melon
  pumpkin
  squash
    acorn
    buttercup

butternut
crookneck
golden nugget
Hubbard
vegetable spaghetti
zucchini
watermelon
Grape family
  brandy
  champagne
  cream of tartar
  grape
  raisin
  wine
  wine vinegar
Grass family
  barley
  barley malt
  bamboo shoots
  bran
  bulgur
  corn
  gluten flour
  graham flour
  hominy grits
  lemon grass
  millet
  molasses
  oat
  popcorn
  rice
  rye
  sorghum
  sugar cane
  triticale
  wheat
  wheat germ
  wild rice
Heath family
  blueberry
  cranberry
  honey

heather
manzanita
huckleberry
Holly family
  maté (yerba maté)
Honeysuckle family
  elderberry
Iris family
  saffron
Laurel family
  avocado
  bay leaf
  cinnamon
  sassafras
Legume family
  alfalfa (sprouts)
  bean
    fava
    kidney
    lima
    mung (sprouts)
    navy
    string
  black-eyed pea
  carob
  chickpea (garbanzo)
  fenugreek
  honey
    alfalfa
    clover
    mesquite
  jicama
  lentil
  licorice
  pea
  peanut
  soybean (lecithin)
  tamarind
Lily family
  aloe vera
  asparagus
  chives

garlic
leek
onion
sarsaparilla
shallot
Madder family
  coffee
Mallow family
  cottonseed oil
  hibiscus
  okra
Malpighia family
  acerola
Maple family
  maple sugar or syrup
Mint family
  basil
  chia seed
  honey
    mint
    rosemary
    sage
    thyme
  horehound
  hyssop
  lemon balm
  marjoram
  oregano
  pennyroyal
  peppermint
  rosemary
  sage
  spearmint
  thyme
Morning Glory family
  sweet potato
Mulberry family
  breadfruit
  fig
  hop
  mulberry

Mustard family
  bok choy
  broccoli
  Brussels sprouts
  cabbage
  cauliflower
  Chinese cabbage
  collards
  honey, cabbage
  horseradish
  kale
  kohlrabi
  mustard greens
  mustard seed
  radish
  rutabaga
  turnip
  watercress
Myrtle family
  allspice
  clove
  guava
Nasturtium family
  nasturtium
Nutmeg family
  nutmeg
  mace
Olive family
  olive
Orchid family
  vanilla
Palm family
  coconut
  date
  sago starch
Papaya family
  papaya
Passion Flower family
  granadilla (passion fruit)
Pedalium family
  sesame seed

Pepper family
  black pepper
  peppercorn
  white pepper
Pineapple family
  pineapple
Pomegranate family
  grenadine
  pomegranate
Potato family
  cayenne pepper
  chili pepper
  eggplant
  paprika
  pepper, sweet
  pimiento
  potato
  tomato
Poppy family
  poppyseed
Protea family
  macadamia nut
Purslane family
  pigweed (purslane)
Rose family
  Pomes
    apple
    crabapple
    honey, hawthorne
    loquat
    pear
    pectin
    quince
    rosehips
  Stone
    almond
    apricot
    cherry
    honey, Hawaiian wild lava
      plum
    nectarine

peach
plum (prune)
Berry
  blackberry
  boysenberry
  dewberry
  honey, raspberry
  loganberry
  raspberry
  strawberry
  wineberry
  youngberry
Sapucaya family
  Brazil nut
Saxifrage family
  currant
  gooseberry
Sedge family
  Chinese water chestnut
  groundnut
Soapberry family
  litchi (lychee)
Spurge family
  cassava
  castor bean
  tapioca (Brazilian arrowroot)
Sterculia family
  chocolate (cacao)
  cocoa
  cocoa butter
  cola nut
Tacca family
  arrowroot, Fiji (Tacca)
Tea family
  tea
Verbena family
  lemon verbena
Walnut family
  black walnut
  butternut
  English walnut

hickory nut
pecan
Yam family
yam

ANIMALS

Mollusks
abalone
clam
cockle
mussel
oyster
scallop
snail
squid
Crustaceans
crab
crayfish
lobster
prawn
shrimp
Fishes (saltwater)
Anchovy family
anchovy
Barracuda family
barracuda
Bluefish family
bluefish
Codfish family
cod (scrod)
haddock
hake
pollack
Croaker family
croaker
drum
sea trout
silver perch
weakfish
Dolphin family

dolphin
Eel family
eel
Flounder family
dab
flounder
halibut
sole
turbot
harvestfish family
butterfish
harvestfish
Herring family
sardine
sea herring
Jack family
pompano
yellow jack
Mackerel family
albacore
bonito
mackerel
skipjack
tuna
Marlin family
marlin
sailfish
Mullet family
mullet
Porgy family
northern scup (porgy)
Scorpionfish family
ocean perch
Sea Bass family
grouper
sea bass
Sea Catfish family
ocean catfish
Swordfish family
swordfish
Tilefish family
tilefish

Fishes (freshwater)
Bass family
  white perch
  yellow bass
Catfish family
  catfish
Croaker family
  freshwater drum
Herring family
  shad
Minnow family
  carp
  chub
Perch family
  yellow perch
Pike family
  pickerel
  pike
Salmon family
  salmon
  trout
Smelt family
  smelt
Sturgeon family
  sturgeon (caviar)
Sucker family
  buffalofish
  sucker
Sunfish family
  black bass
  crappie
  sunfish
Whitefish family
  whitefish

AMPHIBIANS

Frog family
  frog's legs

REPTILES

Alligator family

alligator
Snake family
  rattlesnake
Turtle family
  terrapin
  turtle

BIRDS

Dove family
  dove
  pigeon (squab)
Duck family
  duck
  duck eggs
  goose
  goose eggs
Grouse family
  ruffed grouse (partridge)
Pheasant family
  chicken
  chicken eggs
  pheasant
  quail
  quail eggs
Turkey family
  turkey
  turkey eggs

MAMMALS

Bear family
  bear
Beaver family
  beaver
Bovine family
  beef
  buffalo
  butter
  cheese
  gelatin
  goat

lamb
milk
  buffalo's
  cow's
  goat's
  sheep's
mutton
sheep
veal
yogurt
Deer family
  caribou
  deer (venison)
  elk

moose
reindeer
Hare family
  hare
Opossum family
  opossum
Pronghorn family
  antelope
Squirrel family
  squirrel
Swine family
  hog (pork)
Whale family ·
  whale

Appendix 2

FOODS MOST AND LEAST LIKELY TO CAUSE ALLERGIC REACTIONS

MOST LIKELY

Alcoholic beverages
Apples
Beans
Beef
Cherries
Chicken
Chocolate
Cinnamon
Citrus fruits
Coconut
Coffee
Cola
Corn
Egg white
Fish and shellfish
Garlic
Malt
Melons
Milk and milk products
Mushrooms
Mustard
Nuts
Peanuts
Peas
Pork
Potatoes (white)
Soy
Strawberries
Sugar, beet and cane
Tomatoes
Turkey
Vinegar
Wheat
Yeast

LEAST LIKELY

Apricots
Artichokes
Asparagus
Avocadoes
Barley
Bell peppers, green and red
Buckwheat
Carrots
Chard
Cranberries
Cucumbers
Dates
Egg yolk
Figs
Honey

Lamb
Lettuce
Nectarines
Oats
Parsley
Peaches
Pears
Pepper
Raisins and grapes
Rice
Rye

Squash
Stringbeans
Sugar, maple, and sorghum
Sweet potatoes
Tapioca
Taro root
Vanilla
Veal
Watermelon
Yams

Where to Send for Products

AIR FILTERS

Air Conditioning Engineers. P.O. Box 616, Decatur, IL 62525 (217/692-2812 or 217/422-0311). Activated-charcoal portable room units.

Aireox Research Corporation. P.O. Box 8523, Riverside, CA 92515 (714/689-2981). Activated-charcoal portable room units.

E. L. Foust Company. P.O. Box 105, Elmhurst IL 60126 (312/834-4952). Activated-charcoal portable room and car units.

Clean Air Technology, Inc. 151 University Ave., Suite 205, Palo Alto, CA 94301 (415/324-8020). A variety of air purifiers, including ion generators and air-to-air heat exchangers.

Environmental Purification Systems. P.O. Box 344, Danville, CA 94526 (415/838-2457). Activated-charcoal portable room and car units.

Nigra Enterprises. 12746 Halkirt St., Studio City, CA 91604 (213/506-1495). All types of whole-house filter systems and portable room units including different brands of activated charcoal filters and HEPA filters.

BARRIER CLOTH

The Cotton Place. 2986 Talisman Dr., Dallas, TX 75292 (214/243-4149). Barrier cloth by the yard or in premade zippered mattress covers.

BEAUTY AND HYGIENE

The Body Bar. 1433 Polk St., San Francisco, CA 94109 (415/441-0341). Unscented bath products, hair conditioner, shampoo, soaps.

The Body Shop. 1621 5th St., Berkeley, CA 94710 (415/524-0216). Unscented bath products, lip balms, skin lotions, shampoo; wood combs, natural-clay cosmetics.

Common Scents. 3920A 24th St., San Francisco, CA 94114 (415/826-1019). Unscented bath products, shampoo, soaps.

Nature's Colors. 424 LaVerne, Mill Valley, CA 94941 (415/383-6919). All-natural cosmetics made from clays, natural oils and natural coloring compounds.

The Soap Opera. 38 Miller Ave., Mill Valley, CA 94941 (415/381-0965). Unscented bath products, shampoo, soaps; wood combs.

Vital Life Co. P.O. Box 618, Carlsbad, CA 92008 (714/729-3919 or 714/729-3747). Unscented astringents, cosmetics, hair conditioner.

World of Aloe. 4 Embarcadero Center, San Francisco, CA 94111 (415/421-5588). Unscented cosmetics, skin and tanning lotions.

BEDS

Futons (Japanese folding mattresses, without springs):

Alaya Store and Stitchery. 848 Cole St., San Francisco, CA 94117 (415/731-2681). All-cotton unfireproofed futons with unsprayed batting and unbleached muslin covers.

Futon Designs, Inc. P.O. Box 4092, Dept. B, St. Paul, MN 55104 (612/646-0500). All-cotton futons with unbleached muslin covers. Crib sizes available.

Gentle Wind. 2929 Shattuck Ave., Berkeley, CA 94705 (415/644-1338); 2327 Market St., San Francisco, CA 94110 (415/861-1981); 3267 17th St., San Francisco, CA 94114 (415/863-9696). All-cotton futons. Unbleached muslin covers available by request.

Mary Ann Blair. P.O. Box 1693, Sausalito, Ca 94966 (415/322-0336). All-cotton unfireproofed futons. Will also custom-make futons with customer's own materials.

Shinera. P.O. Box 528, Boston, MA 02102 (800/343-2997). All-cotton futons fireproofed with boric acid. Crib sizes available.

MATTRESSES

Adams Mattress Company. 3804 NE 28th , P.O. Box 7025, Fort Worth, TX 76111 (817/838-2935). All-cotton unfireproofed mattresses made with unsprayed batting. Organic batting available by request.

Community Mattress Company. 1130 Burnett Ave., Concord, CA 94520 (415/798-9785). Will custom-make mattresses from your own materials.

Crown City Mattress. 37 S. Fair Oaks Ave., Pasadena, CA 91101 (213/796-9101 or 213/681-6356). All-cotton unfireproofed mattresses. Unsprayed batting available by request.

Elliot Bedding. 2000 Wright Ave., Richmond, Ca 94804 (415/841-3073). All-cotton unfireproofed mattresses made with barrier-cloth covers by request.

Erlander's Natural Products. P.O. Box 106, Altadena, Ca 91001 (213/797-7004). All-cotton unfireproofed mattresses made with unsprayed batting. Rollaway-bed and crib sizes available.

Janice Corp. 12 Eton Dr., N. Caldwell, NJ 07006 (201/226-7753). All-cotton mattresses. Cotton canvas cots available.

Santa Cruz Mattress & Upholstery Company. 923 Water St., Santa Cruz, CA 95062 (408/426-5073). All-cotton unfireproofed mattresses. Crib sizes available.

Scope Mattress & Pillows. 3576 Stacy Cr. Lumberton, NC 28358 (919/738-8897). All-cotton mattresses fireproofed with boric acid.

BEDDING

Amana Woolen Mills. Amana, IA 52203 (319/622-3432). Unmothproofed wool blankets.

The Atrium. The Anchorage, 2800 Leavenworth, San Francisco, CA 94133 (415/673-5121). Unmothproofed alpaca blankets.

Avoca Handweavers. Ballinacor House, Church Rd., Ballybrack, Co. Dublin, Ireland. Unmothproofed wool bedspreads and blankets.

Cable Car Clothiers/Robert Kirk, Ltd. 150 Post St., San Francisco, CA 94108 (415/397-7733). Cotton afghans; cashmere and viyella blankets.

Clothcrafters. Elkhart Lake, WI 53020 (414/876-2112). Cotton flannel bedlinens.

Conran's. 145 Huguenot St., New Rochelle, NY 10801 (914/632-0999). Patterned cotton percale bedlinens; cotton/down comforters.

The Cotton Place. 2986 Talisman, Dallas, TX 75229 (214/243-4149). Cotton percale bedlinens (crib sizes available); cotton flannel and thermal blankets; cotton felt mattress pads.

Cuddledown. Dept. OG, Main St., Yarmouth, ME 04096 (207/846-5759). Cotton/down comforters.

D. MacGillivray & Co. Muir of Aird, Benbecula, Western Isles, Scotland PA8 85NA. Unmothproofed wool bedspreads and blankets in traditional Scottish highland plaids.

David Morgan. P.O. Box 70190, Seattle, WA 98107 (206/282-3300). Cotton afghans; wool and cotton blankets; crib sizes available.

Day Break. P.O. Box 177, Monterey, MA 01245. Cotton flannel bedlinens in white and colors; cotton blankets.

Eddie Bauer. P.O. Box 3700, Seattle, WA 98124 (800/426-8020). Cotton flannel bedlinens; viyella blankets; cotton/down comforters.

Erlander's Natural Products. P.O. Box 106, Altadena, CA 91001 (213/797-7004). Cotton percale bedlinens (crib sizes available); cotton bedspreads; cotton, unmothproofed wool, and viyella blankets (crib sizes available); cotton/wool comforters; cotton felt mattress pads.

Feathered Friends. Dept. 5, 6 1st Ave., Seattle, WA 98121 (206/622-0974). Flannel bedlinens in white and colors; cotton/down comforters (crib sizes available).

Garnet Hill. P.O. Box 262, Franconia, NH 13580 (603/823-8123). Cotton, cashmere, and wool afghans; cotton flannel bedlinens in white, solid colors, and patterns; wool bedspreads; cashmere, cotton and wool blankets (crib sizes available); cotton/down and cotton/wool comforters.

Homespun Crafts. Dept. RS-2, Box 1776, Blacksburg, SC 29702 (800/458-3491). Cotton afghans and bedspreads.

Icemart. Keflavik International Airport, Iceland. Unmothproofed Icelandic wool blankets.

Janice Corp. 12 Eton Dr., N. Caldwell, NJ 07006 (201/226-7753). Cotton felt mattress pads; cotton/cotton and cotton/wool quilts.

Landau. P.O. Box 671, Princeton, NJ 08540 (800/257-5136). Unmothproofed Icelandic wool blankets (crib sizes available); cotton/Icelandic wool comforters.

Lucy Stewart's Private Stock. P.O. Box 443, Grafton, NH 03240 (603/523-4313). Cotton flannel bedlinens (crib sizes available); cotton bedspreads; cotton and wool blankets.

Norm Thompson. 1805 NW Thurman, Portland, OR 97209 (800/547-1160 or 1532). Cotton afghans; cotton flannel bedlinens in white, solid colors, and patterns.

Old Colony Curtains. P.O. Box 759, Westfield, NJ 07090 (800/526-4298). Cotton beadspreads and blankets.

Orvis. 31 River Rd., Manchester, VT 05254 (802/362-1300). Cotton flannel bedlinens; wool blankets.

Peach Blossom Futon. 3273 Ibis St., San Diego CA 92103 (714/692-0693). Cotton/cotton comforters.

Peruvian Connection. Canaan Farm, Tonganoxie KS 66086 (800/228-2606). Alpaca blankets.

Shinera. P.O. Box 528, Boston, MA 02102 (800/343-2997). Imported cotton percale bedlinens; cotton thermal blankets.

Vermont Country Store. Weston, VT 05161 (802/824-3184). Cotton percale bedlinens; cotton thermal blankets.

Warm Things. 180 Paul Dr., San Rafael, CA 94903 (413/472-2154). Cotton/down comforters.

CELLOPHANE FOOD WRAP

Erlander's Natural Products. P.O. Box 106, Altadena, CA 91001 (213/797-7004).

H. D. Catty Corp. Church & Mills St., Huntley, IL 60142.

Janice Corp. 12 Eton Dr. N. Caldwell, NJ 07006 (201/226-7753).

Nu Vita Food Co. 7524 SW Macadam, Portland, OR 97219.

CLOTHING

A. Garstang & Co. 213 Preston New Road, Blackburn, England BB2 6BP. For men and women. Custom shirts and sleepwear in cotton, silk, and viyella.

After the Stork. P.O. Box 1832, Bisbee, AR 85603 (602/432-3683). For children. Basic cotton clothing.

Banana Republic. P.O. Box 77133, San Francisco, CA 94107 (415/777-5200). For men and women. Cotton outdoor clothes and foreign surplus, authentic safari clothes, cotton windbreakers.

Britches of Georgetowne. P.O. Box 428, Alexandria, VA 22313 (703/548-0200). For men and women. Traditional and outdoor clothing in cotton, linen, silk and wool.

Cable Car Clothiers/Robert Kirk, Ltd. 150 Post St., San Francisco, CA 94108 (415/393-7733). For men and women. Traditional clothing in cashmere, cotton, linen, silk, and wool.

Canterbury Tree. P.O. Box 428, Capistrano Beach, CA 92624. For women. Cotton swimwear.

Carol Brown Putney, VT 05346 (802/387-5875). For women. Custom clothing made with exceptional fabrics from around the world: cotton, linen, silk, unmothproofed wool.

Charing Cross Kits P.O. Box 789, Meredith, NH 03253 (603/279-8449). For women and children. Ready-to-sew clothing kits in unusual English designs.

Chico Pants. P.O. Box 152, Cohasset Stage Route, Chico, CA 95926 (916/342-9178). For women and children. Basic cotton clothing.

Cotton Comfort. 2633 Dalgreen Ct., Plano, TX 75075 (214/867-6418). For men and women. Basic cotton clothing.

Cotton Cookie. 50 Elm Ave., Woodacre, CA 94973 (415/488-0705). For children. Basic cotton clothing.

Cotton Dreams. 999 Laredo Ln., Sebastian, FL 32958 (305/589-0172). For men, women, and children. Basic cotton clothing.

The Cotton Place. 2986 Talisman Dr., Dallas, TX 75229 (214/243-4149). For men, women, and children. Basic cotton clothing.

The Cottonage. 249 Lighthouse, Monterey, CA 93940 (408/373-1795). For children. Basic cotton clothing.

David Morgan. P.O. Box 70190, Seattle, WA 98107 (206/282-3300). For men and women. Cotton and unmothproofed wool outdoor clothing imported from Wales and New Zealand.

Day Break. P.O. Box 177, Monterey, MA 01245. For children. Basic cotton clothing.

Deva Cottage Industry. 303 E. Main St., P.O. Box C, Burkittsville, MD 21718 (301/473-4900). For men and women. Basic cotton clothing in loose-fitting styles.

Dunham's of Maine. Waterville, ME 04901 (800/431-0471). For men and women. Traditional clothing in cotton, linen, silk, and wool.

Erlander's Natural Products. P.O. Box 106, Altadena, CA 91001 (213/797-7400). For men, women, and children. Cotton clothing custom made for Erlander's.

French Creek Sheep & Wool Co. Elverson, Pa 19520 (800/345-4091). For men and women. High-quality sportswear and outerwear made from unmothproofed wool and alpaca, cotton, cashmere, linen, and silk.

Garnet Hill. P.O. Box 262, Franconia, NH 13580 (603/823-8123). For men, women, and children. Imported clothing, sleepwear, and undergarments in cotton, silk, and wool.

Gokey's 84 S. Wabsha St., St. Paul, MN 55107 (612/292-3911). For men and women. Traditional clothing in cotton, silk, and wool.

Good Things Collective, Inc. 52 Main St., Northampton, MA 01060 (413/586-5403). For women. Basic cotton clothing.

Huntington Clothiers. 2258 E. Main St., Columbus, OH 43209 (800/848-6203). For men and women. Traditional clothing in cotton and wool.

Icemart. Keflavik International Airport, Iceland. For men, women, and children. Unmothproofed, undyed Icelandic wool garments.

Irish Cottage Industries, Ltd. 44 Dawson St., Dublin, 2, Ireland. For men, women, and children. Unmothproofed, undyed garments from Ireland.

Jenifer House. Great Barrington, MA 01230 (413/528-1500). For women. Cotton clothing in country styles, including hard-to-find items such as smocks and wedding dresses.

J. Barbour & Sons, Ltd. c/o Guildhall Imports, 40 W. 55 St., New York, NY 10019. For men and women. Egyptian cotton outerwear, waxed for waterproofing.

L. L. Bean. 806 Casco St., Freeport, ME 04033 (207/865-3111). For men, women, and children. Basic cotton clothing.

Landau. P.O. Box 671, Princeton, NJ 08540 (800/257-5136). For men and women. Unmothproofed, undyed Icelandic wool garments.

Land's End. Land's End Ln., Dodgeville, WI 53533 (800/356-4444). For men and women. Outdoor and traditional clothing in cotton and wool.

Orvis. 31 River Rd., Manchester, VT 05254 (802/362-1300). For men and women. Cotton outdoor clothing.

The Peruvian Connection. Canaan Farm, Tonganoxie, KS 66086 (800/228-2606). For men and women. Peruvian imports, unmothproofed by request.

Royal Silk, Ltd. Royal Silk Plaza, 45 E. Madison Ave., Clifton, NJ 07011 (800/621-5559). For women. Silk and silk/cotton clothing.

Victory Shirt Co. 345 Madison Ave., New York, NY 10017 (212/687-6375). For men and women. Cotton shirts.

Vermont Country Store. Weston, VT 05161 (802/824-3184). For men, women, and children. Basic cotton clothing.

FABRICS

A. Garstang & Co. Ltd. 213 Preston New Road, Blackburn, England BB2 6BP. Cotton, silk, viyella.

Conran's. 145 Huguenot St., New Rochelle, NY 10801 (914/632-0999). Cotton.

The Cotton Place. 2986 Talisman Dr., Dallas, TX 75229 (214/243-4149). Cotton and cotton barrier cloth.

D. MacGillivray & Co. Muir of Aird, Benbecula, Western Isles, Scotland PA8 85NA. Cashmere, camel's hair, mohair, unmothproofed wool.

Erlander's Natural Products. P.O. Box 106, Altadena, CA 91001 (213/797-7004). Cotton.

Exotic Silks! 252 State St., Los Altos, CA 94022 (415/948-8611). Cotton and silk.

Gohn Bros. P.O. Box 111, Middlebury, IN 46540. Cotton and wool.

Natural Fiber Fabric Club. Dept. VP 28, 521 Fifth Ave., New York, NY 10175. Cotton linen, silk, wool.

Scotch House. 187 Post St., San Francisco, CA 94108 (415/391-1264); P.O. Box 1983, Orinda, CA 94563 (415/254-4270). Unmothproofed wool and viyella.

Scottish Tartan Shop. 515 Geary St., San Francisco, CA 94102 (415/771-1898). Unmothproofed wool.

Sunflower Studio. 2851 Rd. B1/2, Attn. RS, Grand Junction, CO 81503 (303/242-3883). Cotton, linen, unmothproofed wool, and natural-fiber blends.

Testfabrics, Inc. P.O. Drawer o, 200 Blackford Ave., Middlesex, NJ 08846 (201/469-6446). Untreated, undyed cotton, linen, silk, and wool.

Vermont Country Store. Weston, VT 05161 (802/824-3184). Cotton.

FEMININE PROTECTION

Cycles. P.O. Box 23123, San Jose, CA 95153. Washable and disposable cotton menstrual pads.

FOOD

Ahler's Organic Date and Grapefruit Garden. P.O. Box 726, Mecca, CA 92254 (714/396-2337). Organic dates, grapefruit, and other dried fruits.

Brentwood Exotic Game. 2110 Orange Blossom, San Antonio, TX 78247 (512/494-8706). Wild meats: venison, buffalo, antelope, ram, reindeer, moose, and bear. Other species available by request.

Briggs-Way Co. Ugashik, AK 99683. Alaskan salmon canned in glass.

Colvada Date Co. P.O. Box 908, Coachella, CA 92236 (714/398-3551). Many varieties of organic dates and date products; nuts and dried fruits.

Czimer Foods, Inc. Route 1, Box 285, Lockport, IL 60441 (815/838-3503). Wild meats: pheasant, partridge, guinea, Canadian geese, peacock, quail, squab, duck, venison, buffalo, moose, bear, reindeer, elk, antelope, hippopotamus, lion, caribou, goat, llama, wild boar, and beaver.

Deer Valley Farm. Route 1, Guildford, NY 13780. Bulk organic flours, grains, and beans; organic bakery goods.

Effie May Organic Fruits and Vegetables. Route 1, Box 422B, Alpine, CA 82001 (714/445-2304). Organic produce.

Eiler's Cheese Market. Route 2, DePere, WI 54115 (414/336-8292). Organic cheese.

The Honey Bee Farms. P.O. Box 10, Newport, TN 37821 (615/623-6146). Organic honey.

Jaffe Bros. P.O. Box 636, Valley Center, CA 92082 (714/749-1133). Bulk organic flours and grains, dried fruits, nuts, and seeds.

Quiet Meadow Farm. 8 Quiet Meadow Ln., Mapleton, UT 84663. Organic produce.

Sunburst Farms Natural Foods. 20 S. Kellog, Goleta, CA 93017 (805/964-8681). Wide selection of brand-name packaged foods and organic produce.

Teel Mountain Farm. P.O. Box 83, Stanardsville, VA 22973 (804/985-7746). Organic baby beef and veal.

Timber Crest Farms. 4791 Dry Creeek Rd., Healdsburg, CA 95448 (707/433-2800). Organic dried fruits and nuts.

Vermont Maple Syrup. Brookside Farm, Tunbridge, VT 05077. Maple syrup with no chemical additives.

Vita Green Farms. P.O. Box 878, 1525 W. Vista Way, Vista, CA 92083 (211/714-2163). Organic produce.

Walnut Acres. Penn Creek, PA 17862. Bulk organic flours, grains, dried fruits; organic prepared foods.

PILLOWS (all have cotton covers)

Cuddledown. Dept. OG, Main St., Yarmouth, ME 04096 (207/846-5759). Goosedown/feathers.

Dona Shrier. 825 Northlake Dr., Richardson, TX 85080 (214/235-0485). Organically grown cotton.

Erlander's Natural Products. P.O. Box 106, Altadena, CA 91001 (213/747-7004). Kapok.

Feathered Friends. Dept. 5, 6 1st Ave., Seattle, WA 98121 (206/622-0974). Goosedown/feathers.

KB Cotton Pillow Co. 2704 Echo St., The Woodlands, TX 77380 (713/367-9399). Cotton.

Mary Ann Blair. P.O. Box 1693, Sausalito, CA 94966 (415/332-0336). Cotton or Kapok.

Peach Blossom Futon. 3273 Ibis St., San Diego CA 92103, (714/692-0693). Cotton.

Shinera. P.O. Box 528, Boston, MA 02102 (800/343-2997). Buckwheat hulls.

Warm Things. 180 Paul Dr., San Rafael, CA 94903 (415/472-2154). Duck and goose down/feather.

READING BOXES

Don Scott. Star Route, Eden, TX 76837 (915/869-3013). All-glass custom boxes made to your specifications.

Human Ecology Equipment Design and Fabrication Co. 413 Betty Jo Ln., Garland, TX 75042 (214/494-2946). Reading boxes readymade from a variety of materials.

RUGS AND CARPETS

The Atrium. The Anchorage, 2800 Leavenworth, San Francisco, CA 94133 (415/673-5121). Undyed, unmothproofed alpaca area rugs, readymade or custom made to your own pattern.

Colorado Looms. 1600 Wynkoop, 3rd Flr., Denver, CO 80202 (303/629-9707). Custom handwoven wool area rugs.

Conran's. 145 Huguenot, New Rochelle, NY 10801 (914/632-0999). Cotton area rugs imported from India.

Dellinger. P.O. Drawer 273, Rome, GA 30161 (404/291-7402). High-quality cotton wall-to-wall carpets made of undyed, prewashed yarns without latex backing. Will custom dye to any color.

Erlander's Natural Products. P.O. Box 106, Altadena, CA 91001 (213/797-7004). Cotton area rugs imported from Belgium in oriental designs.

Jenifer House. Great Barrington, MA 01230 (413/528-1500). Wool and wool/cotton area rugs.

Laura Ashley. 1827 Union St., San Francisco, CA 94123 (415/922-7200); Mail Order Dept., 55 Triangle Blvd., Carlstadt, NJ 07072. Cotton area rugs.

SHOWER CURTAINS (cotton)

Clothcrafters. Elkhart Lake, WI 53020 (414/876-2112).

The Cotton Place. 2986 Talisman Dr., Dallas, TX 75229 (214/243-4149).

Erlander's Natural Products. P.O. Box 106, Altadena, CA 91001 (213/797-7004).

Good Things Collective. 52 Main St., Northampton, MA 01060 (413/586-5403).

VITAMINS (all natural)

Advanced Medical Nutrition, Inc. 2575 Buena Vista Ave., Walnut Creek, CA 94596 (415/783-6969). Special Basic Prevention formula to help protect the body from toxic chemicals.

Eden Ranch. P.O. Box 370, Topanga CA 90290. No formaldehyde in gelatin capsules.

Jaffe Bros. P.O. Box 636, Valley Center, CA 92082 (714/749-1133).

Neo-Life. Check phone book for the dealer nearest you. Special Toxguard formula to help protect the body from toxic chemicals.

Nutricology. 2336C Stanwell Circle, Concord, CA 94520. Specially formulated for Type 2 persons.

Seroyal Brands, Inc. P.O. Box 5861, Concord, CA 94524 (415/676-8873).

Vital Life. P.O. Box 618, Carlsbad, CA 92008 (714/729-3919; 729-3747).

Vitaline Formulas. 150 Country Club Dr., P.O. Box 6757, Incline Village, NV 89450 (702/831-5656).

Walnut Acres. Penn Creek, PA 17862.

WATER FILTERS

Bon Del, Inc. P.O. Box 1461, Mesa, AZ 85201 (602/832-3060). Portable plastic charcoal units in countertop and mobile models.

Cactus International Products. P.O. Box 7365, Menlo Park CA 94025 (415/854-7727). Portable plastic charcoal filters in a variety of models and reverse osmosis units.

Environmental Purification Systems. P.O. Box 344, Danville, CA 94526 (415/838-2457). A variety of plastic and all-metal charcoal filters, including a shower-head filter.

Neo-Life Distributors. Check phone book for the dealer nearest you. Plastic charcoal units that attach to the faucet.

YARN

Bartlett Yarns. Harmony, ME 04942 (207/683-2251). Unmothproofed wool.

Belding Lily. P.O. Box 88, Shelby, NC 28150 (704/482-0641). Cotton and wool.

Briggs & Little Woolen Mills, Ltd. York Mills, Harvey Station, York County NB, Canada EoH 1Ho (506/366-5438). Wool.

Brookside Farm. Tunbridge, VT 05077. Unmothproofed and undyed wool.

Cambridge Wools, Ltd. P.O. Box 2572, 16–22 Anzac Ave., Auckland 1, New Zealand. Unmothproofed, undyed wool from New Zealand.

Contessa Yarns. P.O. Box 37, Lebanon, CT 06249 (203/642-7630). Cotton and silk.

The Cotton Place. 2986 Talisman Dr., Dallas, TX 75229 (214/243-4149). Cotton.

Daft Dames Handcrafts. 13384 Hain Rd., Route 5, Akron, NY 14001 (716/542-4235). Cotton, linen, mohair, silk, unmothproofed wool.

Fibers & Fables. 512 S. Mechanic, Pendleton SC 29670 (803/646-9342). Cashmere, linen, silk, unmothproofed wool, and other natural fibers.

Icemart. Keflavik International Airport, Iceland. Unmothproofed Icelandic wool.

Old Mill Yarn. P.O. Box 8, Eaton Rapids, MI 48827 (517/663-2711). Cotton and wool.

Stavros Kouyoumoutzakis. 166 Kalokerinou Ave., Iraklion, Crete, Greece. Unmothproofed, undyed wool.

REFERENCES

TYPE 1 BOOKS

Dehejia, Harsha V. *The Allergy Book*. Chicago: Contemporary Books, 1981.

Frazier, Claude A. *Coping and Living with Allergies*. Englewood Cliffs, New Jersey: Prentice-Hall, 1980.

Giannini, Allan V.; Schultz, Nathan; Chang, Terence T.; Wong, Diane C. *The Best Guide to Allergy*. New York: Appleton-Century-Crofts, 1981.

Knight, Allen. *Asthma & Hayfever*. New York: Arco Publishing, 1981.

TYPE 2 BOOKS

Bell, Iris R. *Clinical Ecology*. Bolinas, Calif.: Common Knowledge Press, 1982.

Dadd, Debra Lynn; Levin, Alan S. *A Consumer Guide for the Chemically Sensitive*. San Francisco: Nontoxic Lifestyles, Inc., 1982.

Golos, Natalie; Golbitz, Frances Golos; Leighton, Frances Spatz. *Coping with Your Allergies*. New York: Simon and Schuster, 1979.

Ludeman, Kate; Henderson, Louise; Basayne, Henry S. *Do-It-Yourself Allergy Analysis Handbook*. New Canaan, Conn.: Keats, 1979.

Mandell, Marshall; Scanlon, Lynne Waller. *5-Day Allergy Relief System*. New York: Pocket Books, 1979.

Newbold, H. L. *Dr. Newbold's Revolutionary New Discoveries About Weight Loss*. New York: Signet, 1979.

Randolph, Theron G.; Moss, Ralph W. *An Alternative Approach to Allergies*. New York: Lippincott & Crowell, 1980.

Travis, Nick; Holladay, Ruth. *The Body Wrecker*. Amarillo, Tex.: Don Quixote, 1981.

COOKBOOKS

Albright, Nancy. *Rodale's Naturally Great Foods Cookbook*. Emmaus, Pa.: Rodale Press, 1977.

Cadwallader, Sharon; Ohr, Judi. *Whole Earth Cookbook*. New York: Bantam, 1972.

Farmilant, Eunice. *The Natural Foods Sweet Tooth Cookbook*. New York: Jove, 1973.

Ford, Marjorie; Hillyard, Susan; Koock, Mary. *The Deaf Smith Country Cookbook*. London: Collier Macmillan, 1973.

Hamrick, Becky; Weiserfeld, S. L. *The Egg-Free, Milk-Free, Wheat-Free Cookbook*. New York: Harper & Row, 1982.

Hewitt, Jean. *The New York Times Natural Food Cookbook*. New York: Avon, 1971.

Hunter, Beatrice Trum. *The Natural Foods Cookbook*. New York: Jove, 1961.

Lappé, Frances Moore. *Diet for a Small Planet*. New York: Ballantine, 1982.

Mandell, Fran Gare. *Allergy-Free Cookbook*. New York: Pocket Books, 1981.

Nasi, Andrea; Rattazzi, Ilaria; Rivetti, Franz. *The Honey Handbook*. New York: Everest House, 1978.

Robertson, Laurel; Flinders, Carol; Godfrey, Bronwen. *Laurel's Kitchen*. New York: Bantam, 1976.

GENERAL

Altman, Nathaniel. *The Chiropractic Alternative*. Los Angeles: Tarcher, 1981.

Biermann, June; Toohey, Barbara. *The Woman's Holistic Headache Relief Book*. Los Angeles: Tarcher, 1979.

Coca, Arthur F. *The Pulse Test*. New York: Arco, 1979.

Eagle, Robert. *Eating and Allergy*. New York: Doubleday, 1980.

Green, Elmer; Green, Alyce. *Beyond Biofeedback*. New York: Dell, 1977.

Kaslow, Arthur L.; Miles, Richard B. *Freedom from Chronic Disease*. Los Angeles: Tarcher, 1979.

Makower, Joel. *Office Hazards*. Washington, D.C.: Tilden Press, 1981.

Rapp, Doris J. *Allergies & Your Family*. New York: Sterling, 1981

Smith, Lendon. *Foods for Healthy Kids*. New York: Berkley, 1981.

Stephenson, Richard M. *Living with Tomorrow*. New York: Wiley, 1981.

Walford, Roy L. *Maximum Life Span*. New York: Norton, 1983.

Index

Abdominal pain, 17, 31. *See also* Gastrointestinal reactions/symptoms
Acquired Immune Deficiency Syndrome (AIDS), 173
Acupressure, 169–170
Acupuncture, 168–169
Ader, Robert, 161–162, 183
Addictions, 18, 97–99, 120–121
  of alcoholics, 118–119
  and chemical sensitivity, 121
  defined, 20
  diagnosis of, 99
  and 5/5 Allergy-Obesity Diet, 123–124
  to foods, 20, 35–36, 96, 97–98
  withdrawal symptoms, 36, 123
Adrenalin, 57, 61, 116, 171
  for insect bite allergy, 56
  pulse test and, 48
  sex and, 171
Affirmation, 166
AIDS (Acquired Immune Deficiency Syndrome), 173
Air filters, 53, 69, 137
  activated carbon, 138–139, 152
  high-efficiency particulate (HEPA), 137
Alcoholism, 118–119
Alkali salts, 78, 79, 87, 116, 124
Allergens
  "conjugated," 181
  defined, 21
  environmental, 33–34, 64, 72, 89–93, 135–147
  Type *1*, 15–16, 20, 35, 42–44
  Type *2*, 15, 20, 36, 71–77, 96, 97–98, 144

Allergic reactions
  and altered homeostasis, 184
  versus nonallergic reactions, 28–32
  See also Type 1 reactions/symptoms; Type 2 reactions/symptoms
Allergic rhinitis, 38, 49–51
Allergies and Your Family (Rapp), 38
Allergists
  clinical ecologists (*see* Clinical ecologists)
  role of, 153
  traditional, 44, 80, 81, 154, 155–156
Allergy/allergies
  defined, 16, 19, 184
  "masked," 98
  origin of term, 19, 183–184
  statistics, 25
  unsuspected, 26
  untreated, 154
Allergy Book, The (Dehejia), 41
Allergy smear, 46
Allpyral shots, 51
Alternative treatments, 161–176
Alupent, 52
Alum-precipitated-allergen, 51
American Academy of Allergy, 95
American Board of Allergy and Immunology, 89
American Lung Association, 39
American Medical Association, 67, 145, 164
Ammonia, 74
Amnesia, 19
Anaphylactic shock, 51, 57, 95, 174
Angioedema, 17, 41
Animal dander/animal hair, 16, 38, 40, 42

Antibodies
  antiidiotypic, 180
  defined, 21, 23
  immunoglobulin E (IgE), 23–24
  monoclonal, 179
Anticaking agents, 101, 108
Antigens
  defined, 21
  effectiveness of, 22
  phenol in, 64
  and provocative-neutralization ther-
    apy, 14, 22, 28, 80–81
  and sexual intercourse, 173
  standardization of, 177
  sublingual, 22, 23, 45, 49–50, 154,
    156
  in testing, 14, 22, 28, 80–81
Antihistamines, 40, 48, 54, 116
  advertising of, 58
  clinical ecologists on, 58
  judicious use of, 59
  side effects, 57, 58–60
  for Type 1 allergies, 57–60
Antiidiotypic antibodies (AIA), 180
Appestat switch-off, 120, 122
Appetite, 17, 19
Applied kinesiology, 81
Arest program, 46
Aroma therapy, 140
Arthritis, 71, 86, 96, 98, 154, 182
Asbestos, 140
Asthma, 16, 37, 38–39
  allergens and, 39
  biofeedback and, 52–53
  cerebral symptoms, 42
  clinical ecology treatments,
    51–53
  conventional treatments, 51–53
  exercise for, 42, 52
  and fluid retention, 39
  and hormonal changes, 39
  and menstruation, 39
  and propranolol, 86
  smoking and, 39
  steroid treatments, 51
  and stress, 39
  and sulfites, 102
  in Type 1 persons, 39
  vitamin C and, 53
Austin, K. Frank, 174–175
Autosuggestion, 166

Backache, 18, 31
Baking powder substitutes, 133
Baking soda, 87, 141
Barrier cloth, 138
Basic Food Sensitivity Diet, 99, 101, 102
  food list A, 104–106
  food list B, 106–107
  purposes of, 103
  recipes, 109–113 (see also Recipes,
    Basic Food Sensitivity Diet)
  sample menus, 108–109
  seven day schedule, 104
  for Type 1 and Type 2 persons, 103
  unprocessed foods as basis for, 103
  and weight loss, 108
B cells, 24, 79, 179
Bedding, 136, 137–138
Bedrooms, removing dust and pollu-
  tants from, 136–139
Bedwetting, 17, 31
Behavioral reactions, Type 2, 64. *See
  also* Cerebral symptoms
Belsky, Marvin, 159
Beverages, 34–35
Beyond Biofeedback (Green and
  Green), 166
Biermann, June, 68
Biofeedback, 53, 162–164
Biological food families, 20, 21, 54, 97,
  104, 193–200
Birth-control pills, 26, 68, 173. *See
  also* Contraceptives
Bjorkland, Anders, 179
Blackouts, 19
Blind tests, 80
Blood cells, 16, 23–24. *See also* B
  cells; T cells
Bodybreather, 52
Bone marrow transplantation, 178–179
Brain
  repair of cell damage, 179
  tumors, 70
  Type 1 reactions, 15
  See also Cerebral symptoms
Breasts, 31
Breathing difficulties, 17, 30–31. *See
  also* Asthma; Bronchitis
Bronchial tubes, in asthma, 38–39
Bronchitis, 39
Buildings, 63, 69, 75. *See also* Pollu-
  tants/pollution: indoor

Burnout, job, 32
Byers, Vera, 54

Cafergot, 87
Calamine lotion, 54
California Medical Clinic for Head-
ache, 68
Cancer, 71, 86, 96, 154
and mononucleosis, 179
skin, 173
visualization and, 167–168
Candida albicans, 76–77, 121, 124
Candidiasus, 31, 76, 115, 136, 137
Candida Food Sensitivity Diet, 100,
115
Cathode ray tube terminals. *See* Video
display terminals (VDTs)
Cardiovascular symptoms, 18
Center for Molecular Nutrition and
Sensory Disorders, 140
Cerebral symptoms, 2, 16, 42, 61, 65
as allergies, 17, 19, 64–71, 72, 177
Challenge testing, 47–48
Food Sensitivity Diets and, 115–117
rotary diet and, 117
Chemicals
avoiding in offices, 146–147
exposure to, 15, 26
immunotoxic, 73–75
removal of, 137–139
Chemical sensitivities, 72–73, 141. *See
also* Type 2 *headings*
conventional allergists and, 155
and compulsive eating, 121
and sugar craving, 121
tests for, 77–82
Chemotherapy
clinical ecologists on, 49
defined, 58
Chest pain, 17, 18, 30
Chicken pox, 41
Chills, 17
Chiropractors, 81, 170–171
Chlorine sensitivity, 74, 75, 101, 174
Chocolate, 37
Cimetidine, 58
Clatton, Lewis B., 39
Cleaners, household, 40
Clinical ecologists, 13–14, 22–23, 37,
64, 78, 89–93
on antihistamines, 58

costs of treatment, 155–156
first office visit with, 156–157
on food allergies, 96
legitimizing of, 155
and lifestyle, 156
points of agreement with traditional
allergists, 154
tests, 45, 80–81
treatments, 22–23, 49–51, 82–93,
154–156
Clothing, 136–137, 138, 142
Coca, Arthur, 19, 48
Coconut milk, 130–131
Cohen, Nicholas, 161–162, 183
Cold sensitivity, 37, 39, 43, 44, 52,
56–57
Colic, in infants, 37
Colitis, 71, 98
Constipation, 18
Contactants, 40, 43, 53–55, 63, 64, 66
Contraceptives, 26, 68, 172, 173
Cooking hints, 130–134
Coping with Your Allergies (Golos and
Golbitz), 54
Corn products, 118–119, 122, 125, 128
Corn-free diets, 133
Cortisone, 51, 52, 54. *See also* Steroids
Cosmetics, 13–14, 40, 43, 141, 142,
172
Costs
of acupuncture, 168–169
of biofeedback treatments, 163
of chiropractic treatment, 171
of hypnosis, 165
of physicians' treatments, 155
See also Medical insurance
Coughs, 17, 30
Cotman, Carl, 179
Coúe, Emile, 166
Cramps
abdominal, 17, 42, 61
menstrual, 18
Cravings. *See* Addictions
Cromolyn sodium, 51–52, 61
Cross-reactions, 97
Cumulative reactions, 20, 96–97
Cytotoxic tests, 27, 46, 79–80

Dancing, 42
Decongestants, 59–61
Dehejia, Harsha V., 41

Depression, 15, 32, 61, 65, 67, 71, 98
  and *Candida albicans*, 76–77
Desensitization treatments, 21, 50–51,
  53
Diagnosis, of Type 1 versus Type 2
  persons, 32–36. *See also* Tests/
  testing
Diarrhea, 17, 31
Diets
  Basic Food Sensitivity Diet, 103–109
  Candida Food Sensitivity Diet, 115
  5/5 Allergy-Obesity Diet, 123–129
  precautionary measures, 100–103
  rules for lasting pattern, 117
  Vegetarian Food Sensitivity Diet,
    114
  See also Cooking hints
Diuretics, 122–123
Dizziness, 17, 70
*Dr. Newbold's Revolutionary New Dis-
  coveries About Weight Loss* (New-
  bold), 172
Doctors. *See* Allergists; Clinical ecolo-
  gists; Physicians
DPOEG, 177
Dracula, 98–99
Drapes, 137
Drugs, 41, 43
  alternatives to, 158
  conventional allergists versus clinical
    ecologists on, 154
  and eczema, 40
  and hives, 41
  prescription, decline in use of, 182–
    183
  questioning physicians on, 158
  Type 1 allergies and, 57–61
Dust, 37, 38, 40, 42
  reduction in home environment,
    136–137
  See also Inhalants

Ears, 15, 16, 17, 18, 29
Eczema, 17, 39, 40, 55
Ecology centers, 27–28, 89
Ecology units, 89–93
  cost of treatment at, 89
  described, 90
  nonallergenic materials in, 91
  treatment at, 90–92
Edema, 18, 118, 122–123

Egg products, 37, 125, 127
Egg-free diets, 131–132
Emotional reactions, 15, 19, 32, 41,
  61. *See also* Cerebral symptoms;
  Depression; Psychosis
Endorphins, defined, 169
Environmental allergens, 64, 72, 89–93
  diagnostic quiz, 33–34
  in home environment, 135–142
  in workplace, 142–147
Environmental control unit. *See* Ecol-
  ogy units
Eosinophils, 46
Epilepsy, 71
EpiPen Auto-Injector, 56, 116
Epoxies, 75
Ergotamines, 87
Estrogens, 68
Ethanol, 14, 81. *See also* Alcoholism
Exercise, 52, 174–175
Eyes, 15, 16, 27–28, 29

Fat, 119–120
Fatigue, 17, 18, 32
Fatty acids, 54–55
Feathers, 43
Fink, Jordan, 174
Fireplaces, 75
5-Day Allergy Relief System (Mandell),
  22
5/5 Allergy-Obesity Diet (AOD), 36,
  100, 123–129
  and fluid retention, 123
  Part 1 (Preparation), 124–125, 126
  Part 2 (Action), 125, 126, 127–129
  reactions to, 123
Fixed reactions, 20, 96
Fluid retention, 18, 39, 118, 122–123
Fluorocarbons, sources of, 75
Flushing, 18
Food additives, 39, 42–43, 67, 96, 101
Food allergies/reactions, 16, 20, 37, 39,
  40, 95–99
  addictive, 20, 35–36, 96, 97–98,
    120–121
  appestat switch-off, 120, 122
  cumulative, 20, 96–97, 116
  edema, 118, 122, 123
  fixed, 20, 96
  and increasing tolerance level, 117
  pulse test for, 19

rotation test for control of, 20, 21
Type 1, 2, 35, 42
Type 2, 2, 36
variable, 20, 96, 97
Food and Drug Administration, 102,
    175, 180
Food containers, 101
Food for Healthy Kids (Smith), 175
Foods, 20–21, 34–36, 61, 68–69, 95–133
    asthma and, 39
    biological families, 20, 21, 193–200
    eczema and, 40
    and exercise, 174
    frozen, 101
    migraine headaches and, 68
    for mold-sensitive persons, 115
    nonallergenic reactions to, 27
    processed, 101, 124–125
    quiz, 34–35
    of similar structure, 20–21
    temperature of, 43
Food Sensitivity Diets (FSD), 36, 99–
    117
    challenge testing, 115–117
    going off, 102
Food Sensitivity Diet (FSD), Basic, 99,
    101, 102, 103–113
    diagnostic purposes of, 103
    foods permitted and excluded from,
    104–105
Food Sensitivity Diets (FSD), Candida,
    100, 115
Food Sensitivity Diets (FSD), Vegetar-
    ian, 100, 114–115
Formaldehyde, 63, 65–66, 73–74, 75,
    140, 178
Fumes, 63, 73–75, 88, 139
    and compulsive eating, 121
    gas, 63, 64, 76, 137, 138
    in offices, 144, 146–147
    paint, 37
    and travel, 150–152
Furniture, 136, 138, 146
Future developments, 177–185

Gall bladder disorders, 71
Gamma-linoleic acid, 54–55
Gardner, Robert W., 20–21
Gas fumes, 63, 64, 76, 137, 138
Gastrointestinal reactions/symptoms,
    17, 42

cimetidine used for, 58
    treatment, 61
    Type 1, 15, 17, 51
    Type 2, 18
Gene therapy, 180–181
Genetic engineering, 179, 180–181
Genetic inheritance, 15, 26, 65
Genitourinary symptoms, 17, 18, 31
Gibbons, Euell, 53
Glycerin preservatives, 77
Goat's milk, 131
Golbitz, Frances, 54
Golos, Natalie, 54
Green, Alyce, 166
Green, Elmer, 166

Halogens, 74
Hamburger, Richard, 25
Harvard School of Public Health, 39
Hay fever, 16, 19, 38
    antihistamines and, 58
    sublingual antigen treatment for, 49–
    51
Headaches
    allergic versus nonallergic types, 29
    versus brain-tumor symptoms, 70
    dull, constant, 70
    location of, 70
    migraine, 15, 19, 67–71
    muscle-spasm or tension, 68, 70, 71
    preventive measures, 87
    sinus, 16, 38, 68
    symptoms, 69–71
    throbbing, 70
Heart
    abnormal rhythms, 18
    disease, 96
Heaters, 137, 138
Heat senstivity, 39, 43, 44, 149
    and eczema, 55
    treatment, 56, 57
    See also Temperature sensitivity
Helper-suppressor ratios, T cell sub-
    sets, 79
Henkin, Robert I., 140
Hepatitis, 41, 65–66, 88
Herbs, 101
Herpes
    genital, 173
    simplex, 41
Hexane, 102

History, of patient, 156–157
Hives, 17, 40, 41
  causative agents, 41, 55
Homeostasis, 184
  defined, 27
  vitamins and, 175
Honey, 130
Hormonal changes, 39
Hormonal imbalance, 121, 169
Horrobin, David, 54
Hotels, 149, 152
House cleaning, 135–142
House dust. *See* Dust; Inhalants
Household cleaners, 40
How to Choose and Use Your Doctor
  (Belsky), 159
Human Ecology Action League
  (HEAL), 136
Humidifiers, 61
Hunger, as allergic reaction, 19, 120–
  121. *See also* Addictions
Hydrolyzed vegetable protein (HVP),
  127
Hyperactivity, 15, 67
Hypersensitivity, 37
Hypnosis, 164–166
Hypothalamus, 122

Iatric Corporation, 46
Idiotypes, 180
IgE. *See* Immunoglobulin E
Immune system, 23–25, 184
  malfunctioning of, 26, 154
immunoglobulin E (IgE)
  in RAST test, 45
  research, 181
  in scratch test, 44
  and T cells, 24–25
  in Type 1 persons, 23–24,
    25
  in Type 2 persons, 24
Immunoglobulin G (IgG), 24
Immunotherapy, 23–25
Immunotoxic chemicals, 73–75
Inderal, 86
Indoor pollutants. *See* Pollutants/pollu-
  tion: indoor
Infants
  Type 1 pattern in, 37
  RAST test for, 46
Infections, avoidance of, 148

Inhalants, 13, 14, 16, 58, 77
  and allergic rhinitis, 38, 50
  and asthma, 39
  and eczema, 40
  and indoor pollutants, 74–76, 135–
    152
  outgassing materials, 74–75
  removal of, 136–137
  and Type 1 allergies, 15, 42
  See also Dust; Pollens; Smoke/
    smoking
Inks, 64, 75, 88, 138
Insect bites, 17, 40, 41, 43, 55–56
  emergency kit for, 56
Insulation of homes, 26
Intal, 51–52
Interferon, 86
Intradermal test, 14, 23, 44, 45, 49, 80
Ions, and video display terminals, 144
Irritability, 17, 61, 65

Jenkins, C. David, 171
Johns Hopkins Allergic Diseases
  Center, 181
Joints, 18, 31, 32
Journals, of food reactions, 100

Kaliner, Michael, 55
Kaposi's sarcoma, 173
Katz, David, 24
Kidneys, and urine autoinjection, 57
Kinesiology, applied, 81
Kudrow, Lee, 68

Lac plant, 54
Lacquer, 54
La Pacho tea, 85
Laughter, inappropriate, 19
Leukemia, 41
Lifestyle, 156
Linoleic acid, 54–55
"Lumpology," 184
Lupus erythematosus, 41, 71, 86

McDevitt, Thomas, 98–99
Mandell, Marshall, 22, 23, 67, 96
Manic depression, 19
Mannitol, 128
Mansfield, John, 68
Medic Alert, 148
Medical insurance, 163, 169

Mediscope, 148
Meditation, 168
Memory loss, 15
Menopause, 68
Menstruation, 18, 39, 68, 71
Menus, Basic Food Sensitivity Diet, 108–109
Metabisulfite, 96
Metal, 40
Metaproteronal sulfate, 52
Micro-Design Systems, 148
Migraine headaches, 15, 19, 67–71
  causes of, 68
  and visual changes, 70
Milk-free diets, 130–131
Milk products, 40, 122–123, 125
  substitutes, 130–131
Mind techniques, 161–168
  affirmation, 166–168
  biofeedback, 162–164
  hypnosis, 164–166
  psychoimmunology, 161–162
Monoclonal antibodies, 179–180
Monoclones, 179
Molds, 16, 37, 39, 42, 115. *See also* Candidiasus; Monilia
Monilia, 115. *See also Candida albicans;* Candidiasus
Monogamy, 173
Monosodium glutamate, 127
Mood changes, 14
Motivation, 153, 173
Mountains, 147
Mouth, dryness of, 18
Mucus, 38–39, 44, 61
Muscles, 18, 31, 32
Muscle test, 81
Mushrooms, 42
Multiple sclerosis, 71, 86, 154

Nasal drops or sprays, 59–60
  saline solution, 60–61
National Aeronautics and Space Administration, 74, 75
National Asthma Center, 52
National Center of Health Statistics, on asthma, 39
National Institute of Allergy and Infectious Diseases, 55, 86
National Institute of Mental Health, 182

National Safety Council, on occupational dermatitis, 145
Natural gas, 63, 64, 76, 137, 138
Natural fibers, 64
Nausea, 17
Neck, 30
Negative ion generators, 144
Neuronotrophic factors, 179
Neutralization, defined, 154. *See also* Provocative-neutralization *headings*
Newbold, H. L., 172
Newsprint, 64, 75, 88, 138
Nonallergenic materials, 91
Nontoxic-living consultants, 136
Nose
  allergy symptoms, 15, 17, 30
  cilia damage, 60
  drops or sprays, 59–61
  and video display terminals, 144
Nut milks, 131
Nystatin, 77, 83

Oat milk, 131
Obesity, 118, 119–123
  5/5 Allergy-Obesity Diet, 36, 100, 123–129
Occupational dermatitis, 145
Occupations, change of, 145
Odors, 13–14, 63–64, 138–142
  chemical, 138
  sensitivity to, 18
  See also Fumes
Offices, pollutants in, 143–147
Oils, cold-pressed, 102
Orthomolecular therapy, 175
Outgassing, 73, 144
  from electric blankets, 137
Overweight, 18, 36. *See also* Obesity

Paint, 37, 76, 139
Patient's right to know, 157–159
Pasteur, Louis, 72
Penicillin, 178
Perfume, 40, 64, 139. *See also* Cosmetics; Odors
Personality changes, 15
Pesticides, 101, 102
Petrochemicals, 73
Pets, 137. *See also* Animal dander/ animal hair

Pharmacokinetics, 183
Phenols, 14, 65–66, 88, 97, 101
Phenylephrine, 60
Phenylpropanolamine (PPA), 59
Phenyls, 21
Phobias, 65–66
Photocopiers, 142, 143, 144, 146
Physicians
   choice of, 152–160
   costs, 155
   family, 153–154, 155
   questioning, 157–158
   See also Allergists; Clinical ecologists
Pirquet, Clemens von, 19
P-N. *See* Provocative-neutralization
   headings
Pneumonia, recurrent, 30
Poison ivy and poison oak, 40, 53, 54
Pollens, 16, 38, 39, 42, 58. *See also* Inhalants
Pollutants/pollution, 26, 38, 72, 88, 89
   effects on T cells, 24
   indoor, 26, 75–76, 135–152
Polyesters, 72, 73, 75
Polyethylenes, 75
Polypropylene, 72
Polystyrene, 101
Polyurethanes, 72, 73, 75, 101
Polyvinyls, 72, 75
Potassium metabisulfite, 95, 102
Premenstrual tension, 18
Preservatives, 101, 102
Primrose oil, 54–55
Processed foods, 101, 124–125
Propanolol, 86
Prostaglandin E (PGE), 55
Provocative-neutralization (P-N)
   intradermal test, 23, 45, 49, 80
   sublingual test, 14, 22, 28, 80–81
   therapy, 22, 23, 45, 49–50, 154 (*see also* Sublingual antigens)
Psychoneuroimmunology (PNI), 161–162
Psychosis, 19, 23, 24, 65, 81. *See also* Cerebral symptoms; Schizophrenia
Pulse Tach Fingertip Heart Computer, 48
Pulse test, 19, 48

Radiation, 143–144, 158
Radioallergosorbent test (RAST), 45–46, 79

Radon, 140
Randolph, Theron, 22, 67, 118
Rapp, Doris, J., 38
RAST. *See* Radioallergosorbent test
Rea, Bill, 90–91
Reading boxes, 90, 138
Rebound phenomenon, 60
Recipes, Basic Food Sensitivity Diet, 109–113
   Cabbage Cauliflower Salad with Raisins, 111–112
   Duck with Ginger Orange Glaze, 110
   Lentil Soup, 113
   Millet Dressing with Currants, 111
   Roasted Yams, 110
   Roquefort Walnut Salad, 111
   Sauteed Chicken with Limes, 112
   Sesame Broccoli, 110
   Spearmint Snow, 112
   Spinach Salad with Lemon Pepper Dressing, 109
Regulatory system, 184
Resins, 76
Respiratory symptoms, 16–17
   Type *1*, 15, 16–17
   Type *2*, 18
Restaurants, 102
Rhinitis, allergic, 38, 49–51
   sublingual antigen treatment for, 49–51
   See also Hay fever
Rhinitis medicamentosa, 60
Rinkel, Herbert, 19–20
Robinson, Ben, 60–61
Rogers, Malcolm, 162
Rotation diet, 20, 28, 88, 102
   biological food families as basis for, 20, 21
   and challenge testing, 117
Rowe, Albert, 19
Runners, breathing devices for, 52
Rush Therapy, 50–51

Saifer, Phillis, 90–91
Salt, 39, 108
   nasal irrigation solution, 60–61
Scents. *See* Odors
Schizophrenia, 19, 66, 71, 77
Scratch tests, 21–22, 44
Scripps Clinic and Research Foundation, 95, 102

Seashore, 147
Seasonings, natural, 108
Seed milk, 131
Seizures, convulsive, 19, 179
Self-healing, 153
Semen, allergy to, 172, 173
Sex therapy, 171–173
Sexual intercourse, 173
Sheep's milk, 131
Sheffer, Albert L., 175
Shellfish, 37
Silicons, 75
Simonton, Carl, 167
Simonton, Stephanie, 167
Sinus problems, 16, 38, 68
Skin reactions/symptoms, 17, 53–55
    itchiness, 17, 32
    occupational dermatitis, 145
    Type 1, 15, 17, 40–41
    Type 2, 18
Smith, Lendon, 175
Smith, Michael O., 169
Smoke, smoking, 39, 40, 65, 137, 138,
    140–141, 145, 146
Sniff test, 78–79
Social mores, 26
Society for Clinical Ecology (SCE), 90–
    91, 93, 155
Sodium bicarbonate, 87, 141
Sorbitol, 128
Soy milk, 131
Speizer, Frank E., 76
Spohn, Richard, 140
Staphylococcus aureus, 41
Steroids, 48–49, 181
    in decongestants, 60
    future treatments, 181
    ointment, 55
    side effects, 60
    See also Cortisone
Stevenson, Donald D., 95
Stress, psychological, 76, 116, 171
    asthma and, 39
    reduction, 171
Strom, Terry, 162
Sublingual antigens, 22, 23, 45, 49–50,
    154. *See also* Provocative-neutral-
    ization *headings*
Sublingual tests, 14, 22, 28, 80–81
Sugar, addiction to, 118, 121, 124
Sugar-free diets, 130
Sulfiting agents, 102

Sulfur, 101
Sulfur dioxide, 74
Sullivan, Timothy J., 177–178
Sunlight, and hives, 41
Surgery, and allergies, 37
Sweating, 18
Sweeteners, 130
    diet, 128
Swimming, 40, 43, 52, 56, 174
Symptoms. *See* Allergic reactions; Type
    1 reactions/symptoms; Type 2 re-
    actions/symptoms
Synthetic compounds and materials,
    63, 66, 69, 71–75, 91, 121, 137.
    See also Chemicals

Tagamet, 58
T and B cell count and helper/suppres-
    sor ratios T cell subsets, 79
Tartrazine, 42
T cells, 16, 23
    in asthmatics, 51
    count, 79
    deficiencies, 23–24
    functions of, 24
    and immunoglobulin E, 24–25
    and immunotherapy, 24
    and interferon, 86
    Rush Therapy and, 50
    in Type 1 persons, 23
    urine autoinjection and, 57
    and visualization, 167
Technicians, 158–159
Television sets, 90
Temperature sensitivity
    and asthma, 52
    and hives, 41
    and swimming, 52
    treatment, 56–57
    and Type 1 allergies, 43–44, 148
Tepes, Prince Vlad, 98–99
Terpenes, 76
Tests/testing
    allergy smear, 46
    Arest program, 46
    blind, 48
    challenge, 47–48, 115–117
    by conventional analysts, 44, 154–
        155
    cytotoxic, 27, 46
    at home, 27, 47–48, 78–79
    intradermal, 14, 23, 44, 45, 49, 80

in laboratory, 45–46, 79–80
in office, 44–45, 80–82
provocative-neutralization (*see under*
  Provocative-neutralization)
pulse, 48
radioallergosorbent (RAST), 45–46
scratch, 21, 44
sublingual, 14, 22, 28, 80–81
for Type 1 allergies, 44–48
for Type 2 allergies, 77–82
Therapies. *See* Treatments
Thirst, excessive, 19
Thymosin, 86
Tobacco Institute, 39
Tobacco smoke. *See* Smoke/smoking
Togo, Africa, 72
Tolerance threshold, defined, 16
Toohey, Barbara, 68
Total load
  defined, 66
  reduction of, 80
Traditional allergists. *See* Allergists:
  traditional
Transfer factor, 86, 92, 178
Transportation, 149, 150–152
Travel, 147–152
Treatments
  acupressure, 169–170
  acupuncture, 168–169
  affirmation, 166
  for allergic rhinitis, 49–51
  alternative, 161–176
  antigen therapy, 82–85
  antihistamines, 57–59
  for asthma, 51–53
  biofeedback, 162–164
  body techniques, 168–176
  chiropractic, 170–171
  choice of, 25
  of clinical ecologists, 22–23, 49–51,
    82–93, 154–156
  for cold and heat sensitivity, 56–57
  conventional, 48–49
  decongestants, 59–61
  at ecology units, 89–93
  exercise, 174–175
  future developments, 178–181
  for hay fever, 49–51
  hypnosis, 164–166
  for insect bites, 55–56
  interferon, 86

intravenous sodium bicarbonate, 87
La Pacho tea, 85
limitations of, 85
mind techniques, 161–168
need for, 152–153
nystatin, 83–84
propranolol, 86–87
provocative-neutralization, 22, 23,
    45, 49–50, 154
psychoneuroimmunology (PNI), 161–
    162
sex therapy, 171–173
for skin disorders, 53–55
stress reduction, 171
sublingual antigens, 22, 23, 45, 49–
    59, 154
Thymosin, 86
transfer factor, 86, 92, 178
for Type 2 persons, 82–87
urine autoinjection, 57
visualization, 167–168
vitamins, 175–176
Tropical and Geographical Magazine,
    53
Truss, C. Orian, 76
Type 1 allergens, 15, 16, 42–44
  food, 20, 35, 96–98
  testing for, 44–48
  and Type 2 reactions, 15, 19
Type 1 persons, 63
  affirmation treatments for, 166
  B cells, 23–24
  bedrooms of, 136–137
  case study, 63–64
  clothing, 142
  and conventional allergists, 155
  defined, 15
  diagnostic quiz, 32–36
  depression, 67
  example of, 37–38, 63–64
  exercise, 174
  and hotels, 149–150
  portrait of, 37–62
  and provocative-neutralization ther-
    apy, 23
  and restaurants, 148
  and sexual intercourse, 171
  T cells, 23, 24
  transportation, 149
  versus Type 2, 25, 32–36
  workplace, 145–146

Type 1 reactions/symptoms, 15, 16–19,
  38–42
  and aging, 42
  asthma, 39
  cerebral, 42, 61
  and cigarette smoke, 145
  cross-reactions, 97
  cumulative food reactions, 97
  diminishment with time, 62
  drug treatments, 57–61
  eosinophils, 46
  first appearance, 15
  fixed food reactions, 96
  gastrointestinal, 42, 61
  inheritance of, 15
  and immunoglobulin E, 23–24, 25
  to insect bites, 41
  to scratch tests, 21
  skin disorders, 40–41
  systemic, 17, 38–42
  target organs, 15
  to temperature changes, 148
  treatments, 48–62
  and Type 2 allergens, 15, 19
Type 2 allergens, 15, 71–77, 144, 145
  food reactions, 20, 36, 96, 97–98
  and Type 1 reactions, 15, 19
Type 2 persons, 92
  affirmation treatments for, 166
  and alcoholism, 118–119
  bedrooms of, 137–139
  clothing, 142
  defined, 2, 15
  depression in, 67
  diagnostic quiz, 32–36
  exercise, 174
  hotels and, 152
  immunoglobulin E in, 24
  and obesity, 118, 119–123
  provocative-neutralization therapy
    for, 23
  and restaurants, 148
  and sexual intercourse, 172
  and travel, 150–152
  versus Type 2, 25, 32–36
  and vitamins, 176
  workplace, 146–147
Type 2 reactions/symptoms, 15, 18–19,
  63–71
  brain cell damage, 179
  conventional allergists on, 154

cross-reactions, 97
  and fat, 119–120
  first appearance, 15
  future treatments, 181
  headaches, 67–71
  and immunoglobulin G, 24
  to insect bites, 41
  research on treatment of, 181, 182
  systemic, 18
  T cells, 24
  testing for, 77–82
  treatments, 82–87
  and Type 1 allergens, 15, 19
Tyramine, 68

Universal reactors, 32, 87–93
  and brain cell damage, 179
  defined, 25
  diagnostic quiz, 32–36
  example of, 87–89
  improvement of, 88, 93
  potential to become, 117
Urination, 17, 31
Urine autoinjection, 57
Urticaria. *See* Hives
Urushiol, 40, 53–54
  antibody injections for reactions to,
    54
  in lacquer, 54
  transmission of, 40

Vacations, 147
Vacuum cleaners, 137
Vaginal yeast infections, 31, 76–77,
  115, 136, 137
Variable reactions
  defined, 20
  to food, 96, 97
Vaughn, Warren, 20, 21
Vegetarian Food Sensitivity Diet, 114–
  115
Ventilation systems, 26
Vertebrae, alignment of, 170
Video display terminals (VDTs), 143–144
Virus infections, 15, 21, 76
  social mores and, 26
Vision
  allergic versus nonallergic symptoms,
    29
  blurred, 27–28
  and migraine headaches, 70

Visualization, 167–168
Vitamin A, 61, 176
Vitamin B, 56, 176
Vitamin C, 79, 116, 124, 175, 176
Vitamins, 92, 175–176
  binders in, 176
Vomiting, 17

Walking, 52
Water, 101
Weather changes, 68
Weight
  fluctuation, 18
  formula for determining, 120
  gain, 18, 36
  See also Obesity
Wheals, 14, 21, 41
Wheat products, 125, 127
  addiction to, 118
Wheat-free diets, 132–133
Wheezing, 17

Williamson, Bob, 181
Wine, 74, 95
Withdrawal symptoms, 36, 123
Wood, 76
Wool, 43
*Woman's Holistic Headache Relief Book,
  The* (Biermann and Toohey), 68
Workplace
  allergies associated with, 142–147
  change of, 145
  pollutants in, 26, 142–147

X-rays, records of, 158

Yeast-free cooking, 133
Yeast infections, 76–77
Yeast products, 115, 125, 128–129
  addiction to, 118
Yoga, 168

Zen Buddhism, 168